*Illustrated Cases in
Acute Clinical Medicine*

For Churchill Livingstone

Publisher: Laurence Hunter
Project Editor: Dilys Jones
Copy Editor: Lesley J. Knott
Design: Design Resources Unit
Production Controller: Debra Barrie
Sales Promotion Executive: Marion Pollock

Illustrated Cases in Acute Clinical Medicine

K. C. McHardy MD MRCP (UK)
Lecturer, Department of Medicine and Therapeutics, University of Aberdeen

D. J. Godden MD MRCP (UK)
Lecturer, Department of Medicine and Therapeutics, University of Aberdeen

D. Nathwani MB ChB MRCP (UK) DTM&H
Senior Registrar, Royal Infirmary, Aberdeen

Gillian Needham BSc MB BCh FRCR
Consultant Radiologist, Royal Infirmary, Aberdeen

K. P. Duguid FBIPP, FRPS, HonFIMI
Director, Department of Medical Illustration, University of Aberdeen

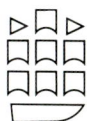

CHURCHILL LIVINGSTONE
EDINBURGH LONDON MADRID MELBOURNE NEW YORK AND TOKYO 1994

CHURCHILL LIVINGSTONE
Medical Division of Longman Group UK Limited

Distributed in the United States of America by Churchill Livingstone Inc., 650 Avenue of the Americas, New York, N.Y. 10011, and by associated companies, branches and representatives throughout the world.

Text © Longman Group UK Limited 1994
Illustration © Grampian Health Board 1994

All rights reserved. No part of this publication may be reproduced, stored in a retrieval system, or transmitted in any form or by any means, electronic, mechanical, photocopying, recording or otherwise, without either the prior permission of the publishers (Churchill Livingstone, Robert Stevenson House, 1–3 Baxter's Place, Leith Walk, Edinburgh, EH1 3AF), or a licence permitting restricted copying in the United Kingdom issued by the Copyright Licensing Agency Ltd, 90 Tottenham Court Road, London, W1P 9HE.

First published 1994

ISBN 0-443-04697-2

British Library Cataloguing in Publication Data
A catalogue record for this book is available from the British Library.

Library of Congress Cataloging in Publication Data
Illustrated cases in acute clinical medicine/K.C. McHardy...
   [et al.].
      p.   cm.
   Includes index.
   ISBN 0-443-04697-2
   1. Internal medicine -- Case studies.   I. McHardy, K.C.
   [DNLM: 1. Clinical Medicine -- case studies.   2. Critical Care -- case studies.   WB 105 I29 1994]
RC66.144 1994
616' .09 -- dc20
DNLM/DLC
for Library of Congress   93-14398
                                                       CIP

The publisher's policy is to use paper manufactured from sustainable forests

Printed in Hong Kong
LYP/01

Contents

Introduction   vii
Acknowledgements   ix
Abbreviations   xi
Laboratory reference ranges   xii

SECTION 1
Case histories   1

1. Breathlessness and ankle swelling   2
2. Abdominal pain/swelling   4
3. Fever, malaise   7
4. Headache, right-sided weakness   9
5. Breathlessness   12
6. Diarrhoea and vomiting   15
7. Abdominal pain, collapse   17
8. Haematemesis   20
9. Breathlessness, weight loss   22
10. Chest pain   25
11. Breathlessness, anaemia   27
12. Sore throat, rash   29
13. Chest infection, drowsiness   31
14. Dysphagia   33
15. 'Blackouts'   35
16. Tiredness, anaemia   37
17. Fit   39
18. Jaundice   41
19. Collapse, diarrhoea   43
20. Drug overdose   45
21. Dysuria/loin pain   47
22. Jaundice, weight loss   49
23. Wheeze, breathlessness   51
24. Bloody diarrhoea   54
25. Abdominal pain, weight loss   56
26. Breathlessness, pallor   58
27. Chest pain   60
28. Breathlessness, abdominal pain   62
29. Right-sided weakness   64
30. Sweats, weight loss   66
31. 'Off her legs'   68
32. Swollen neck   71
33. Headache   73
34. Breathlessness   75
35. Chest pain, breathlessness   78
36. Jaundice/abdominal pain   80
37. Thirst/polyuria   82
38. Abdominal pain   84
39. Chest pain   86
40. Swelling   88
41. Collapse   90
42. Shingles   92
43. Headaches, collapse   94
44. Vomiting blood   96
45. Painful foot   98
46. Night sweats, tiredness   100
47. Chest pain   102
48. Collapse, ? fit   105
49. Breathlessness   107
50. Backache, weak legs   109

SECTION 2

Self-assessment exercises 113

1. MCQs 114
2. MCQ answers 117
3. Quiz questions 119
4. Quiz answers 122

Index 123

Introduction

It is difficult to learn clinical medicine at the bedside without some knowledge of the contents of medical textbooks; it is impossible to learn clinical medicine in the library. This collection of case histories makes an attempt, insofar as a book can, at bridging the gap between the theory and practice of clinical medicine. The cases are all based on real patients with personal details altered to preserve anonymity, and some factual details amended to improve clarity or utilize an educational opportunity.

The presentation, as in the real-life situation on an acute medical ward, is problem based; the receiving board announces the reason for admission as 'breathlessness', or 'headache and vomiting' or 'collapse' and not as a diagnosis of asthma, subarachnoid haemorrhage or Stokes–Adams attacks. The challenge (as in clinical practice), is to use the information presented on history, examination and investigation results to arrive at the correct diagnosis. In addition to textual and numerical data, a wide range of illustrative material has been used to display the visual clues provided by physical signs, radiological and non-radiological investigations, and bedside record charts.

Without any deliberate attempt at misleading obscurity, some items of extraneous historical material are included to encourage a healthy discriminatory attitude to the analysis of clinical data. Similarly, the 'routine investigation results' include a great deal of information which, as in the real situation, is available but may make no positive contribution to the diagnostic process. Explanatory notes are given on how the findings led to the final diagnosis and, where appropriate, why possible alternative diagnoses were rejected. Every effort has, however, been made to avoid the all-inclusive style of more formal textbooks, which necessarily sacrifice readability for comprehensiveness.

Notes on therapeutic and prognostic outcome, provided for completeness, are brief, for this is not a textbook of medical treatment. Key pieces of information summarizing the main points for each case will facilitate learning and aid revision. The self-assessment section, which includes a number of cross-referenced items relating to different cases exhibiting common features, is based exclusively on the contents of the book.

We hope that this book will entertain, educate and encourage the less experienced diagnostician by increasing confidence in the recognition of patterns of clinical information. Anyone who can confidently deal with the 50 different diagnostic scenarios presented here is well on the way to coping efficiently with 'solving' his or her next 50 acute medical diagnostic problems.

K.C.McH.
D.J.G.
D.N.
G.N.
K.P.D.

Aberdeen 1994

Acknowledgements

We would like to acknowledge the help of the following colleagues in the compilation of material for this book: Dr P.D. Bewsher, Dr Joanne Currie, Dr R.J.L. Davidson, Mr A. Dick, Dr J.G. Douglas, Dr J.A.R. Friend, Sister Maggie Grundy, Dr P.W. Johnston, Dr C.R. Levi, Dr Mary McKean, Dr H. McKenzie, Dr A.W. McKinlay, Dr N.A.G. Mowat, Dr J.C. Patel, Dr S. H. Ralston, Mr I.W. Reid, Dr Olive Robb, Dr G.B. Scott, Mr G. Sinton and Dr C.C. Smith. We are particularly grateful to Dr Giles Roditi for his assistance with the collection of radiological material.

We would also like to thank the many colleagues who discussed the material included in the book for their helpful suggestions and Professor J.C. Petrie for his encouragement. Finally, we are grateful to the staff of the Department of Medical Illustration of the University of Aberdeen, and to those patients who gave permission for their photographs to be reproduced here.

K.C. McH.
D.J.G.
D.N.
G.N.
K.P.D.

Abbreviations

The use of abbreviations is a widespread and economical phenomenon in medical practice – provided the reader is familiar with the abbreviation used! We have used this book as an opportunity to introduce the reader to several commonly used abbreviations by giving the full name of the relevant item where it first appears in a chapter followed by the popular abbreviation in parentheses. In some cases, particularly in relation to the routine investigation panel, the abbreviations are not explained for reasons of space. These abbreviations and a number of others which appear throughout the text are explained below:

AAT	aspartate aminotransferase
Alb	albumin
AP	alkaline phosphatase
APTT	activated partial thromboplastin time
Bil	bilirubin
Cr	creatinine
CSF	cerebrospinal fluid
CT	computerized tomography
ECG	electrocardiograph
ESR	erythrocyte sedimentation rate
γGT	gamma glutamyl transpeptidase
Glu	glucose
Hb	haemoglobin
HCO_3	bicarbonate
HIV	human immunodeficiency virus
Ig	Immunoglobulin
K	potassium
Ke	ketones
MBq	megaBecquerel
MCV	mean corpuscular volume (erythrocytes)
Na	sodium
neg	negative
NSAID	non-steroidal anti-inflammatory drug
Plt	platelets
Pr	protein
PT	prothrombin time
SpG	specific gravity
tr	trace
TSH	thyroid stimulating hormone
T3	triiodothyronine
T4	thyroxine
U	urea
WCC	white blood cell count

Laboratory reference ranges

The laboratory reference values given in this book generally follow the customary convention of including the 95% confidence interval for values for apparently healthy individuals studied using the particular methods employed in the local laboratory. Reference values are often very similar in different laboratories but should never be regarded as being universally applicable due to the different methodologies and different 'normal populations' in different geographical locations.

For investigation results reported only occasionally throughout the book, reference ranges have been given alongside the individual results. For the 'routine investigations' and blood gases the reference values are given below, and are not repeated elsewhere.

Biochemistry
serum Na 137–144 mmol/l
serum K 3.5–4.9 mmol/l
serum HCO_3 22–30 mmol/l
serum Urea 3.4–7.0 mmol/l
serum Creatinine 60–110 µmol/l
serum Albumin 37–49 mmol/l
serum Bilirubin 1–22 µmol/l
serum Aspartate aminotransferase 5–31 U/l
serum Alkaline phosphatase 45–105 U/l
serum Gamma glutamyl transpeptidase 5–35 U/l

Haemotology
Haemoglobin male 140–180 g/l; female 120–160 g/l
Mean corpuscular volume 82–99 fl
White cell count 4.0–10.0 x 10^9/l
Platelet count 150–400 x 10^9/l
Erythrocyte sedimentation rate 0–15 mm at 1 hour

Blood gases
Values given in the book relate to arterial blood gases. Oxygen and carbon dioxide partial pressures are given in kiloPascals (kPa). The abbreviation $sHCO_3$ stands for 'standard bicarbonate' which relates to the bicarbonate concentration in a sample held at a standard pCO_2 (5.3 kPa) to separate metabolic from respiratory disturbances of acid–base balance. Reference values in our laboratory are:

pH 7.35–7.42; pO_2 10.6–13.3 kPa;
pCO_2 4.5–6.0 kPa; $sHCO_3$ 21–25 mmol/l

Urinary specific gravity
The concept of a reference range is not altogether applicable to urinary specific gravity. Its value can vary greatly in different situations and its utility lies in its relationship to prevailing conditions. It should simply be remembered that a urine with a specific gravity of 1.010 (or approximately 290 mOsm/kg) is isosmotic with plasma. Dilute urine (SpG < 1.010) results from loss of water in excess of solute, and concentrated urine (SpG > 1.010) from loss of solute in excess of water.

Section 1
Case histories

The main part of this book consists of 50 individual case histories, with each patient presented in a similar format, as an emergency admission to a general medical ward. The title gives the patient's name and age, and principal reasons (symptoms or signs) for referral. The history of the presenting complaint is followed by notes on previous medical history, family and social history, and drug therapy. The examination findings are described, then a table of routine investigation results (biochemistry, haematology and urinalysis) is followed by a series of additional results of tests peculiar to the case in question. The next section summarizes the case and reveals the diagnosis, explaining how it was reached, and why possible alternatives were rejected. There then follow some brief notes on the outcome for the patient. Finally, a series of key points has been prepared (under the headings of history/examination, investigations, and outcome) for the purposes of emphasis and easy revision.

Grace Woolley (88)
Breathlessness and ankle swelling

CASE HISTORY

Mrs Woolley had felt increasingly tired and breathless on exertion for 2 months prior to presentation. She had developed ankle swelling, which improved temporarily when her general practitioner prescribed a diuretic, but subsequently recurred despite a doubling of the dose. She noted progressive generalized weakness and was latterly having difficulty in even rising from a chair. Despite a reasonable appetite, she had lost around 6 kg in weight and her bowels had been loose. On enquiry, she denied having chest pain but had been aware of a fluttering sensation in her chest. She had a dry cough, which was worse while lying in bed. There were no other symptoms of note.

There was no past medical history. A brother had died of rheumatic fever in his thirties, and another of heart disease at 80 years. Mrs Woolley neither smoked nor drank alcohol. She lived independently in sheltered accommodation with assistance from her daughter who lived nearby.

EXAMINATION

She looked frail and lean with diffuse thinning of her hair (Fig. 1.1). She was mildly dyspnoeic at rest. There was pitting oedema at both ankles but no mucosal pallor. Her hands were warm and moist and there was a fine tremor of her outstretched fingers. Her pulse was irregular at about 130/min, and blood pressure was around 170/70. There was an ejection systolic murmur at the cardiac base, which radiated into the neck and was audible over a firm, nodular swelling in her neck (Fig. 1.1) that she said had been present, unchanged, for over 40 years. The jugular venous pressure was raised. The percussion note was dull at the right lung base and fine inspiratory crepitations were heard over both lung fields. Abdominal examination was unremarkable. The tendon jerks were all rather brisk, and there was some weakness of proximal muscles.

INVESTIGATIONS

Routine investigation results

Urine	SpG 1.012	Pr tr	Glu neg	Ke neg	Blood neg
Serum	Na 137	K 3.8	HCO_3 27	U 8.4	Cr 57
	Alb 37	Bil 6	AAT 14	AP 119	γGT 25
Blood	Hb 130	MCV 80	WCC 6.4	Plt 262	ESR 15

Additional investigations

An electrocardiogram (ECG) (Fig. 1.2) and chest radiograph (Fig. 1.3) were as illustrated. Thyroid function tests showed a total T4 of 228 nmol/l (reference range 70–150), free T3 of 19.0 pmol/l (3–9) and thyroid-stimulating hormone (TSH) by immunoradiometric assay of <0.1 mU/l (0.35–3.3). Antimicrosomal and antithyroglobulin antibodies were not detected in serum.

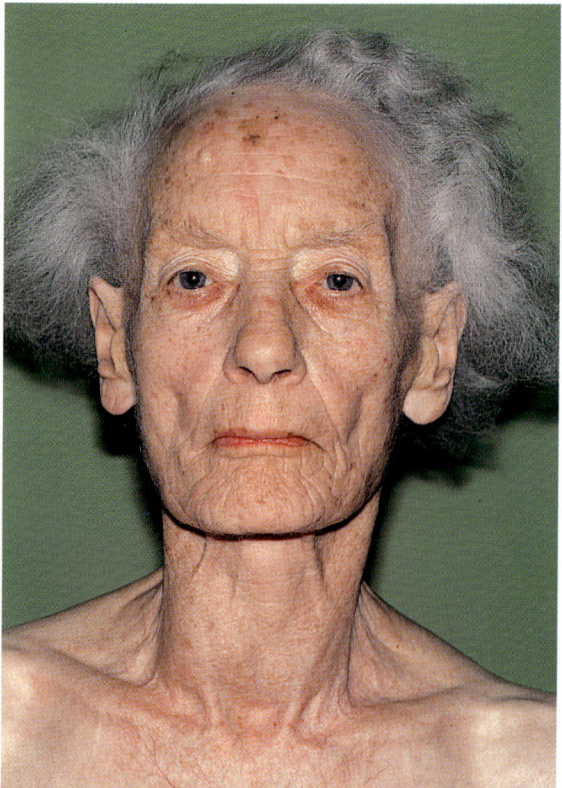

Fig. 1.1
Appearances of face and neck.

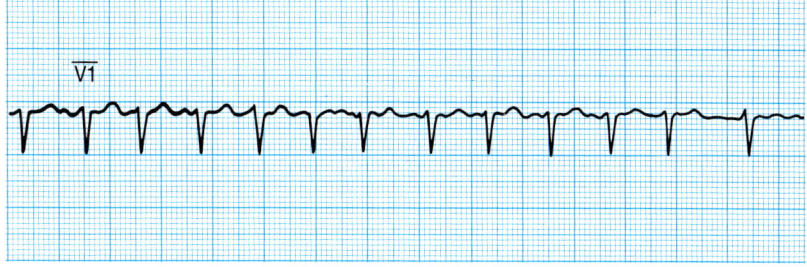

Fig. 1.2
ECG (lead V1) showing tachycardia of approximately 150/min and features of atrial fibrillation (irregularly irregular QRS complexes and absence of P waves).

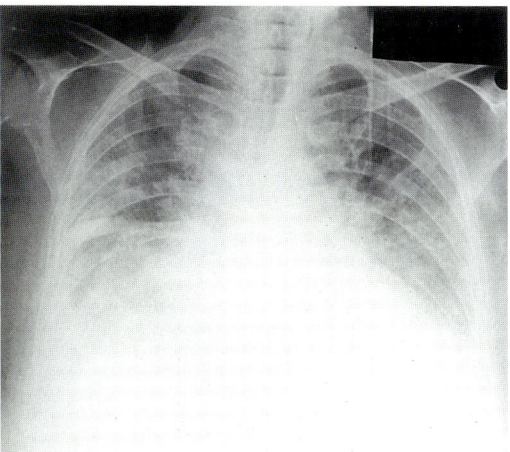

Fig. 1.3
Chest radiograph showing cardiomegaly, pulmonary oedema and pleural fluid at the right base and in the horizontal fissure.

DIAGNOSIS

Mrs Woolley had cardiac failure complicating hyperthyroidism. The latter was suggested by the combination of weight loss, tremor, palpitations, diarrhoea and muscle weakness, and was confirmed by the high thyroid hormone levels and suppressed TSH. The clinical appearances of the thyroid gland indicated that she had a toxic multinodular goitre (rather than Graves' disease in which the thyroid gland is usually smooth and there may be associated ophthalmopathy). Cardiac complications were indicated by the ECG findings (fast atrial fibrillation) and chest radiograph (pulmonary oedema, right basal effusion and fluid in the horizontal fissure).

The presentation with breathlessness, weakness and exhaustion is typical in elderly patients with hyperthyroidism; although most of the classical features are present, the diagnosis is often less obvious than in younger patients. The systolic bruit heard over the thyroid was not necessarily of diagnostic importance as it may have simply been a conducted aortic sclerotic murmur. This patient's long history of goitre and short history of hyperthyroid symptoms serve to emphasize that thyroid size and function are frequently unrelated.

OUTCOME

Mrs Woolley responded quickly to treatment with loop diuretic, beta-blocker and digoxin. Anticoagulation was considered but not implemented in view of her age and frailty. She received a therapeutic dose (370 MBq) of ^{131}I and her thyroid function tests returned to normal within 3 months. She was managing to live independently at the time of her 90th birthday. She was clinically and biochemically euthyroid at that time, and her goitre remained unchanged. Provision was made for periodic thyroid function testing in view of the substantial risk of post-radioiodine hypothyroidism and requirement for thyroxine replacement therapy.

KEY POINTS

History/Examination
- Remember thyrotoxicosis as a cause of cardiac failure in the elderly.
- The clinical appearances of the thyroid gland are not always a guide to its function.

Investigations
- Suspicion of thyroid dysfunction is necessary in order that appropriate investigations are requested.
- Clinical features of thyrotoxicosis are often non-specific and biochemical confirmation is essential.
- The combination of elevated thyroid hormones (especially free hormones) and suppressed TSH is typical of hyperthyroidism.

Outcome
- The treatment of cardiac failure resulting from hyperthyroidism can be very successful, even in frail, elderly patients.

2 Robert Hay (62)
Abdominal pain/swelling

CASE HISTORY
Mr Hay, a lorry driver, presented with a 3-month history of intermittent, dull, aching central abdominal pain. During this time, he had noticed that his abdomen was swelling, such that he had bought larger trousers. He had been lethargic and his appetite was poor. He had also noted ankle swelling during the previous month, although he had lost about 3 kg in weight. He was breathless on exertion, e.g. while mowing his lawn.

He had a history of a duodenal ulcer diagnosed 2 years previously, and of diphtheria in childhood. He lived with his wife in a two-storey house. He smoked 20 cigarettes daily and for many years had drunk a substantial amount of alcohol, admitting to about 20 pints of beer and 10 whiskies per week.

EXAMINATION
He looked unwell and had generalized muscle wasting. He had white nails (leuconychia) (Fig. 2.1) and palmar erythema (Fig. 2.2). There were widespread spider naevi over his face and upper chest (Fig. 2.3) and he had gynaecomastia and testicular atrophy. He was not jaundiced. His pulse was 80/min, blood pressure was 130/80 and his heart sounds were normal. He had bilateral pitting ankle oedema. There was dullness to percussion and reduction in breath sounds and vocal resonance at the right lung base posteriorly. His abdomen was distended, and percussion revealed shifting dullness. The liver was palpable 2 cm below the costal margin, but the spleen was not palpable. There was no neurological abnormality.

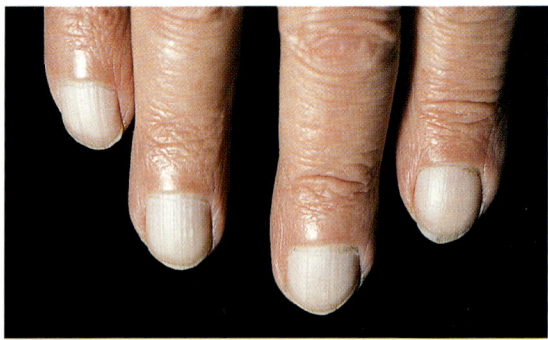

Fig. 2.1
White nails – leuconychia.

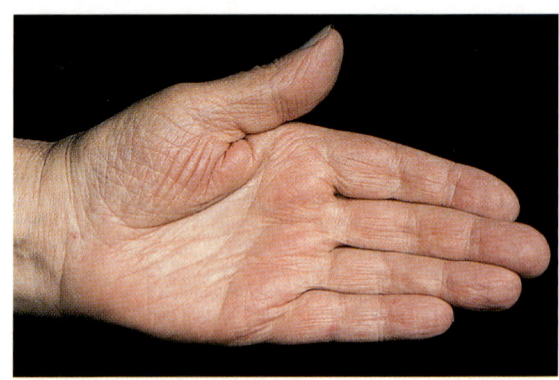

Fig. 2.2
Palmar erythema.

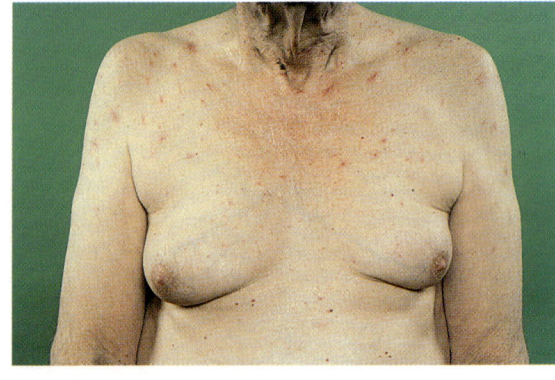

Fig. 2.3
Appearances of the upper chest showing multiple spider naevi and gynaecomastia.

INVESTIGATIONS
Routine investigation results

Urine	SpG 1.005	Pr tr	Glu neg	Ke neg	Blood neg
Serum	Na 134	K 4.3	HCO₃ 28	U <2	Cr 63
	Alb 23	Bil 12	AAT 39	AP 186	γGT 95
Blood	Hb 137	MCV 99	WCC 7.1	Plt 200	ESR 26

Additional investigations

Hepatitis B surface antigen was negative. A clotting screen showed PT 15.9 s (reference range 12–16), APTT 39.5 s (35–45) and TCT 16.4 s (12–17). Numerous round macrocytes and stomatocytes were seen on the blood film. Serum alpha-fetoprotein was 5 µg/l (reference range 0–25), serum copper 23 µmol/l (15–25) and serum ferritin 339 µg/l (20–350). Smooth muscle antibody, antimitochondrial antibody and antinuclear antibody were negative.

His chest radiograph was abnormal (Fig. 2.4). An abdominal ultrasound scan (Fig. 2.5) showed hepatomegaly with an irregular echo pattern in the liver, and confirmed the presence of ascites. A liver biopsy showed distortion of the liver architecture with the presence of fibrous septa and regenerative nodules.

DIAGNOSIS

The history and clinical findings, together with the low blood urea and albumin, abnormal liver enzymes and blood film appearances, indicate that this man has chronic liver disease. The long history of high alcohol intake is the most likely cause, and the liver biopsy features confirm that he has cirrhosis. The clinical findings indicate that he now has portal hypertension and ascites, the latter due partly to a combination of portal hypertension and hypoproteinaemia. The hypoproteinaemia in this condition is predominantly related to impairment of albumin synthesis in the damaged liver and may also reflect poor dietary protein intake. The chest radiograph shows a right pleural effusion which is most likely due to transdiaphragmatic leak of ascitic fluid. Other possible causes of cirrhosis were considered but are unlikely in view of the negative additional investigations: chronic active hepatitis (smooth muscle antibody), primary biliary cirrhosis (antimitochondrial antibody), haemochromatosis (serum ferritin), Wilson's disease (serum copper) and biliary obstruction (ultrasound scan).

Patients with alcoholic cirrhosis are at increased risk of developing hepatocellular carcinoma, which can be detected by ultrasound scanning and may be associated with an elevated serum alpha-fetoprotein.

Mr Hay had no clinical evidence of portosystemic encephalopathy, which is a neuropsychiatric syndrome associated with shunting of blood from the portal to the systemic circulation. Clinical features to suggest this include impaired conscious level, a flapping tremor of the outstretched hands, difficulty in performing manual tasks such as drawing complex shapes (constructional apraxia), and in severe cases, coma with hyper-reflexia and extensor plantar responses.

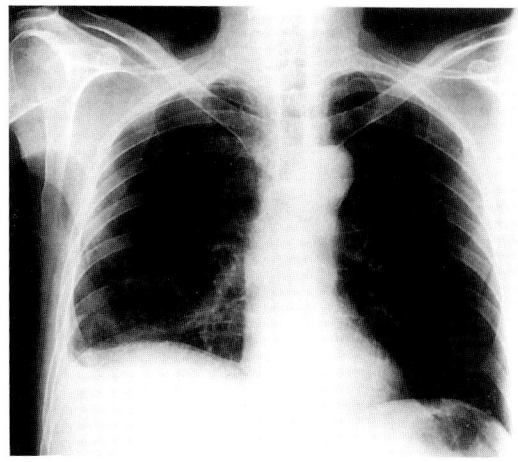

Fig. 2.4
Chest radiograph showing a small right pleural effusion.

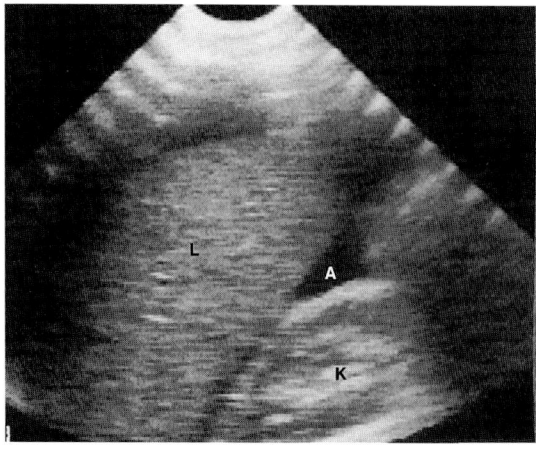

Fig. 2.5
A right parasagittal ultrasound section through the upper abdomen showing the right lobe of liver (L), right kidney (K) and ascites (A).

OUTCOME

He was treated with bed rest and modest doses of diuretics, and his ascites gradually resolved. At review 2 months later, he was abstinent from alcohol, and was feeling well. The ascites had resolved, his serum albumin had risen to 34 g/l and his blood urea to 2.7 mmol/l. The γGT, alkaline phosphatase and AAT levels had reduced though remained above the reference range.

KEY POINTS

History/Examination
- Excessive alcohol intake is the commonest cause of cirrhosis in Europe and North America.
- Liver function can be severely impaired without the presence of jaundice.

Investigations
- The association of low serum urea and albumin, deranged liver enzymes and round macrocytosis is suggestive of chronic liver disease.
- Liver disease may be associated with impaired clotting and thrombocytopenia, which may preclude liver biopsy.
- In patients with cirrhosis, a high serum alpha-fetoprotein is suggestive of the coexistence of hepatocellular carcinoma.

Outcome
- In alcoholic liver disease, some recovery of hepatic function may be possible if the patient remains abstinent from alcohol.

John McKay (32)
Fever, malaise

CASE HISTORY
John McKay, a veterinary surgeon, had been vaguely unwell for 2 months before being admitted to hospital for investigation. He described tiredness and shortness of breath with recurrent episodes of sweating and shivering.

Three years earlier a routine medical examination had detected a cardiac murmur. He was referred for cardiac catheterization, which had revealed mild aortic regurgitation. He remained well until 4 months before this admission, when he had noticed haematuria and had undergone cystoscopy. This was performed as an outpatient and was normal. He had received no medication during the course of his illness.

He had previously undertaken occasional trips to Kenya where he was involved in tuberculin testing of cattle but his most recent trip had been more than 6 months ago. He was married with two children. He was a non-smoker and drank alcohol socially.

EXAMINATION
He was pale, clammy and unwell with a fever of 38.3°C. Lesions were present under the finger and toe nails (Fig. 3.1). His pulse was 110/min, regular and collapsing and blood pressure was 140/60. Auscultation of the praecordium revealed an early diastolic murmur, maximal at the left sternal edge. Both lung bases had scattered crepitations. Abdominal and neurological examinations were normal.

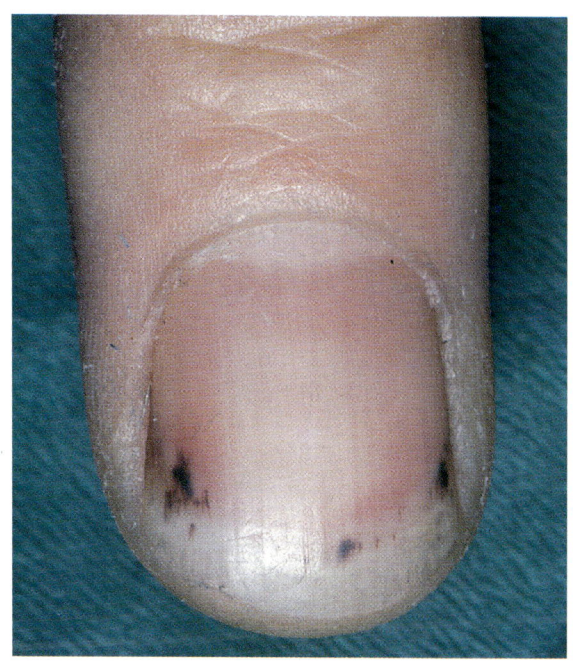

Fig. 3.1
Appearances of finger nail.

INVESTIGATIONS
Routine investigation results

Urine	SpG 1.001	Pr tr	Glu neg	Ke neg	Blood +++
Serum	Na 130	K 3.7	HCO$_3$ 20	U 6.7	Cr 123
	Alb 25	Bil 7	AAT 40	AP 30	γGT 10
Blood	Hb 90	MCV 89	WCC 16.7	Plt 400	ESR 57

Additional investigations

C-reactive protein (CRP) was elevated at 9 mg/dl (reference range <1). The chest radiograph and ECG were within normal limits. Blood cultures revealed a growth of *Streptococcus faecalis*. A two-dimensional echocardiogram was performed (Fig. 3.2).

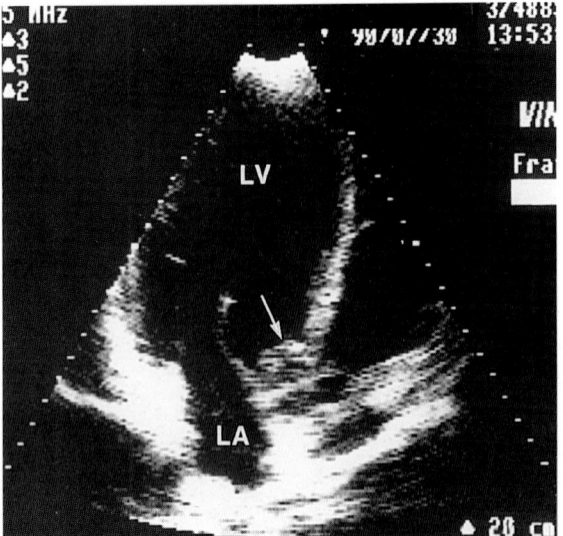

Fig. 3.2
Apical four-chamber echocardiographic view showing the left ventricle (LV) and left atrium (LA). There are vegetations on the aortic valve (arrow).

DIAGNOSIS

Recurrent fever associated with sweating, malaise and shivering is indicative of episodic bacteraemia, and the classic triad of features of infection, underlying valvular heart disease and splinter haemorrhages (Fig. 3.1) suggests the diagnosis of bacterial endocarditis. Recent use of invasive genitourinary instrumentation without prior antibiotic prophylaxis was responsible for the introduction of *Strep. faecalis*. The murmur of aortic regurgitation was heard, but in bacterial endocarditis murmurs often change during the course of the illness. Haematuria occurs in association with bacterial endocarditis and is due to either glomerular emboli or an immune-complex-mediated nephritis.

OUTCOME

Mr McKay was treated successfully with high doses of intravenous antibiotics. He subsequently required repeat cardiac catheterization and aortic valve replacement.

KEY POINTS

History/Examination
- In a patient with pre-existing valvular heart disease who develops a fever, infective endocarditis must be considered.
- A congenital bicuspid aortic valve is the commonest underlying cardiac abnormality.

Investigations
- The isolation of *Strep. faecalis* from the blood confirms the clinical diagnosis.
- A normochromic, normocytic anaemia, low serum albumin, fast ESR and raised CRP reflect chronic sepsis.
- In infective endocarditis, echocardiography reveals vegetations in about 60% of patients.

Zeinab Patel (41)
Headache, right-sided weakness

CASE HISTORY
Mrs Patel had recently returned from a shopping trip when she suddenly fell to the floor complaining of a very severe pain in the left side of her head behind her eye. She retched a few times but did not vomit. Her husband noticed that her face appeared twisted, and as she tried to get up, her right leg seemed to give way under her. She became drowsy and her speech was strange and unintelligible. The general practitioner was called and sent her to hospital, his referral letter adding that she was previously well with no significant past medical history. There was no family history of note; she was not taking any medication and smoked 10 cigarettes per day.

EXAMINATION
On admission she was a little restless but breathing regularly. She opened her eyes when spoken to, but her attempts at verbal response were limited and made no sense, although they included some clearly recognizable words. She had a right-sided facial weakness and there were no spontaneous movements of her right arm or leg. The pupils were equal and reacting to light. The optic discs were normal but there was an extensive subhyaloid haemorrhage in the left eye (Fig. 4.1). The gag reflex was intact, and there was mild neck stiffness. Tone was reduced in the right-sided limbs and the right plantar response was extensor. Her pulse was 70/min and blood pressure was 188/104. The chest and abdomen were clinically normal.

INVESTIGATIONS
Routine investigation results

Urine	SpG 1.011	Pr neg	Glu neg	Ke neg	Blood neg
Serum	Na 137	K 3.9	HCO$_3$ 25	U 4.8	Cr 69
	Alb 38	Bil 16	AAT 25	AP 92	γGT 24
Blood	Hb 13.8	MCV 85	WCC 9.3	Plt 272	ESR 9

Additional investigations
A CT scan of the head showed blood distributed throughout the subarachnoid space (Fig. 4.2). A chest radiograph showed normal heart size and clear lung fields, and an ECG showed sinus rhythm with normal complexes and, in particular, no evidence of left ventricular hypertrophy. Internal carotid artery digital

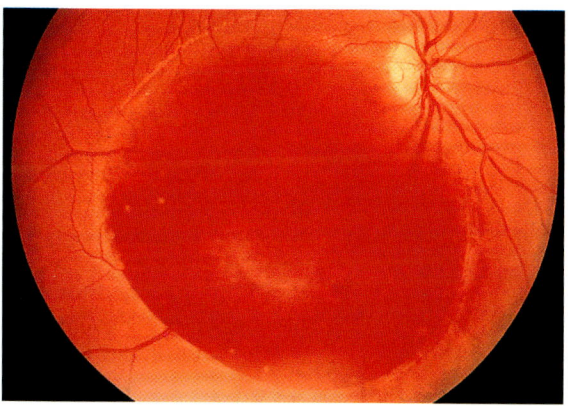

Fig. 4.1
Fundoscopic appearances showing subhyaloid haemorrhage covering the macular region.

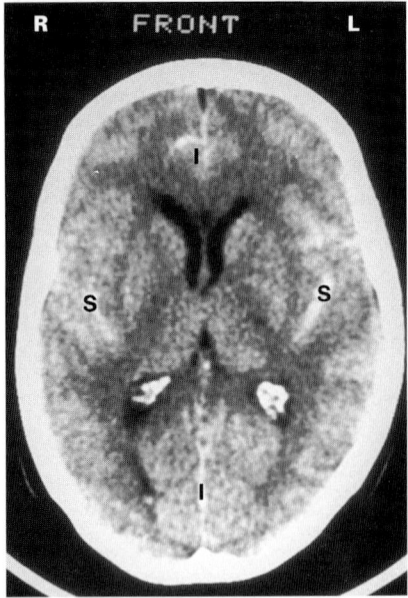

Fig. 4.2
Single transverse CT section through the head at the level of the lateral ventricles showing blood in the Sylvian fissures (S) and in the interhemispheric fissure (I).

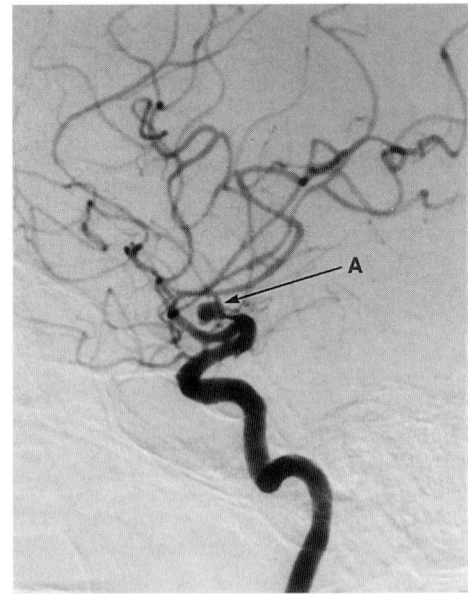

Fig. 4.3
Single film from an angiographic series showing aneurysm (A).

subtraction angiography showed an aneurysm of the left anterior communicating artery (Fig. 4.3); the other major vessels were normal.

DIAGNOSIS

Mrs Patel had suffered a subarachnoid haemorrhage resulting from rupture of a berry aneurysm on the left anterior communicating cerebral artery. The sudden onset of severe headache with signs of a right hemiparesis were highly suggestive of this diagnosis. The development of neck stiffness was due to meningeal irritation caused by blood in the cerebrospinal fluid (CSF); this may take several hours to develop. There were no other features suggestive of meningitis in this case. A subhyaloid haemorrhage may be seen following the acute rise in intracranial pressure resulting from an intracranial haemorrhage. The pattern of neurological deficit suggests a problem in the left cerebral cortex. The speech difficulty was dysphasia, a disorder of language (comprehension and/or production) occurring as a result of ischaemia in the dominant cerebral hemisphere. The clinical diagnosis of intracranial haemorrhage was quickly confirmed by CT head scanning. Lumbar puncture at this stage may have shown blood-stained CSF, but this investigation is best avoided if head scanning facilities are available owing to the slight risk of cerebral coning following lumbar puncture in the presence of raised intracranial pressure. Cerebral angiography confirmed the nature of the underlying lesion and gave important information on its exact location and orientation. Hypertension at presentation is a common acute phenomenon; there were no features of sustained hypertension on fundoscopy, chest radiography or electrocardiography.

OUTCOME

Mrs Patel's restlessness abated and her conscious level returned to normal. Her speech improved greatly over a few days. She was treated with analgesics and the cerebral vasodilator, nimodipine. She proceeded to craniotomy 8 days after presentation, when the aneurysm was exposed and its neck successfully clipped. After 2 months of inpatient rehabilitation, her speech was near normal and she was able to manage independently despite a residual right hemiparesis.

KEY POINTS

History/Examination
- A very severe headache of sudden onset with or without associated neurological deficit is highly suggestive of an intracranial bleed, the commonest spontaneous cause being rupture of a berry aneurysm causing subarachnoid haemorrhage.
- Neck stiffness is a common finding where there is subarachnoid blood but it may take several hours after the haemorrhage to develop.

Investigations
- An early CT head scan is the investigation of choice where available. Following a small bleed or if presentation is delayed by a day or more, the CT scan may appear normal, in which case lumbar puncture should be performed to look for CSF xanthochromia (discoloration due to the presence of blood pigment).
- If there is any doubt that a patient is suffering from meningitis, lumbar puncture is an essential early investigation.
- Cerebral angiography is necessary to define the source of haemorrhage (and to look for similar lesions elsewhere on the cerebral circulation).

Outcome
- Without surgical intervention the risks of rebleeding are very high. Opinion varies on the optimal time for surgery but most would advocate intervention within 10 days if the patient's general condition permits.
- The prospects for neurological recovery are better in younger patients, with lesser initial deficits; recovery is often incomplete although a substantial proportion of cases do not develop a neurological deficit at any stage.

Charles Smith (65) Breathlessness

CASE HISTORY
Mr Smith, a widower, had developed increasing breathlessness and wheeze, and was breathless at rest for 48 h before admission. He was coughing up green sputum, but no blood. His ankles had been swollen during the previous week. He had noticed breathlessness on heavy exertion, such as climbing stairs, for several years. For the previous 4 years, he had also suffered a cough productive of white sputum occurring most mornings.

He denied previous illnesses, and had been employed as a fish processing worker until 60 years of age, when he was made redundant. He smoked 40 cigarettes daily and drank 10 units of alcohol per week. He was not taking medication, apart from an occasional antacid tablet for heartburn.

EXAMINATION
He was drowsy, but orientated in place and time, and was pyrexial (37.8 °C). His tongue and fingers were cyanosed, but he had warm peripheries and a coarse flapping tremor of the outstretched hands. His pulse was 130/min, and jugular venous pressure was raised to the level of the ear lobe (Fig. 5.1). The second heart

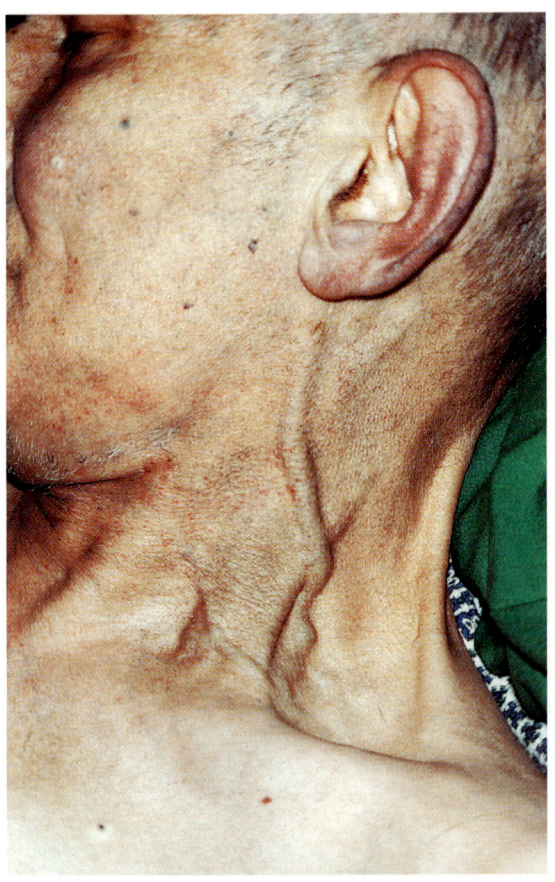

Fig. 5.1
Lateral view of the neck showing elevation of the jugular venous pressure and cyanosis visible in the ear.

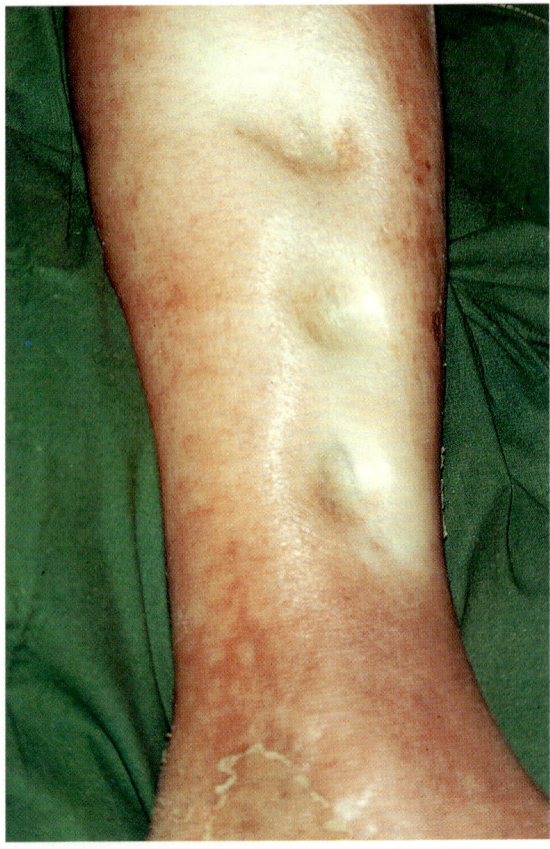

Fig. 5.2
View of the ankle showing pitting oedema.

sound was loud and there was bilateral pitting ankle oedema (Fig. 5.2). His respiratory rate was 32/min, the chest was hyperinflated and he was using accessory muscles of respiration. The breath sounds were vesicular with a prolonged expiratory phase, and bilateral expiratory wheezes were present. There were coarse crackles audible over the left lower chest posteriorly. His liver edge was palpable 3cm below the costal margin, but the spleen was not palpable. There were no focal neurological abnormalities and the optic fundi were normal.

INVESTIGATIONS
Routine investigation results

Urine	SpG 1015	Pr neg	Glu neg	Ke neg	Blood neg
Serum	Na 140	K 4.5	HCO_3 39	U 6.3	Cr 74
	Alb 31	Bil 8	AAT 22	AP 82	γGT 18
Blood	Hb 180	MCV 81	WCC 12.2	Plt 327	ESR 22

Additional investigations
The haematocrit was 0.55 l/l (reference range 0.34–0.51) and the red cell count was $5.8 \times 10^{12}/l$ ($4-5 \times 10^{12}/l$). Arterial blood gases (breathing air) were as follows:

pH	pO_2	pCO_2	$sHCO_3$
7.31	3.1	9.1	28.0

The sputum contained pus cells and a significant growth of *Haemophilus influenzae* on culture. The ECG (Fig. 5.3) and chest radiograph (Fig. 5.4) were both abnormal.

DIAGNOSIS
The diagnosis is of an acute infective exacerbation of chronic obstructive airways disease. Flapping tremor and warm cyanosed extremities are clinical signs of carbon dioxide retention. The blood gas results show severe hypoxia and hypercapnia, which confirm that he had ventilatory failure, and the clinical signs of right heart failure indicate cor pulmonale (i.e. right heart failure secondary to primary lung disease).

Despite his claim of only mild symptoms prior to the current illness, the productive cough suggests chronic bronchitis. The chronic nature of his disease is also suggested by the elevated serum bicarbonate, indicating renal compensation for a chronic respiratory acidosis, and by his ability to tolerate severe hypoxia without more pronounced neurological impairment.

He also had evidence of secondary erythrocytosis, with elevated haemoglobin, haematocrit and red cell count, as a result of chronic hypoxia.

The ECG (Fig. 5.3) shows right axis deviation and tall peaked P waves (P pulmonale), suggesting pulmonary hypertension, which had been suspected clinically by the presence of a loud second heart sound. Hyperinflation of the lung fields on chest radiography is indicated by the fact that the posterior ends of more than 10 ribs are visible above the diaphragm.

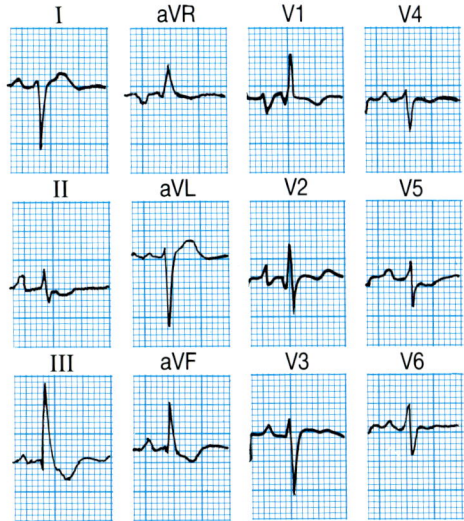

Fig. 5.3
ECG showing right axis deviation and P pulmonale.

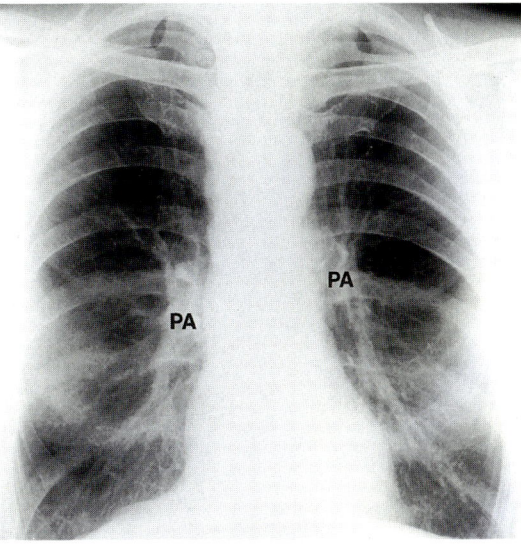

Fig. 5.4
Chest radiograph showing hyperinflation of the lungs and prominent pulmonary arteries (PA).

OUTCOME

Mr Smith was treated initially with 24% oxygen, nebulized bronchodilators, intravenous antibiotics and oral diuretics, and made a gradual improvement. The arterial pCO_2 fell to 7 kPa, without resort to a respiratory stimulant.

Pulmonary function tests were performed in the recovery phase and showed typical features of obstructive airways disease, with a reduction in the peak flow and FEV/FVC ratio and an increased residual volume indicating intrathoracic gas trapping. The transfer factor for carbon monoxide (tCO) was also reduced, indicating loss of diffusing capacity in the lungs due to the presence of emphysema.

He was encouraged to stop smoking, but over the following year his pulmonary function declined and he died 14 months later with a further exacerbation of symptoms.

KEY POINTS

History/Examination
- Acute deterioration in a patient with chronic obstructive airways disease may be precipitated by infection.
- Drowsiness and a flapping tremor are signs of carbon dioxide retention. Papilloedema may also occur.

Investigations
- The combination of hypoxia and hypercapnia indicates ventilatory failure.
- Elevation of the standard bicarbonate in association with ventilatory failure indicates renal compensation.

Outcome
- During oxygen therapy in patients with chronic hypoxia and hypercapnia, it is important to monitor arterial pO_2 and pCO_2, since administration of excess oxygen may depress ventilation leading to worsening acidosis.

Tracey McIntosh (21)
Diarrhoea and vomiting

CASE HISTORY
Miss McIntosh, an agriculture student, presented to the Emergency Department in the early hours of the morning complaining of a few hours' history of severe vomiting. She had 'cramping' abdominal pain and frequent loose watery motions but no dysuria. About 30 h earlier, she had gone out with friends for a meal to celebrate the end of term and afterwards had had three pints of lager. On the day prior to admission, she had been well and had spent much of the morning horse riding. Her flatmate, who accompanied her to hospital, had shared the celebration meal and was also complaining of diarrhoea and vomiting, though her symptoms were less severe.

Miss McIntosh had not recently travelled abroad. She smoked 10 cigarettes daily and drank moderate amounts of alcohol regularly. She was not taking medication, except for the oral contraceptive pill. She lived in a flat with three other students. In view of her condition, she was admitted to the Infection Unit.

EXAMINATION
On admission, she appeared mildly dehydrated and was febrile (38.5 °C). Her pulse was 84/min, blood pressure 120/80 and there was no postural drop in blood pressure. Abdominal examination revealed slight epigastric abdominal tenderness and increased bowel sounds. There was tenderness on rectal examination and the stool was negative for occult blood. The remainder of the examination was normal.

INVESTIGATIONS
Routine investigation results

Urine	SpG 1.020	Pr neg	Glu neg	Ke +	Blood neg
Serum	Na 140	K 4.2	HCO$_3$ 29	U 5.1	Cr 78
	Alb 42	Bil 3	AAT 16	AP 56	γGT 19
Blood	Hb 133	MCV 81	WCC 12.3	Plt 248	ESR 10

Additional investigations
Blood cultures were negative. Stool cultures grew *Salmonella enteritidis* (Fig. 6.1).

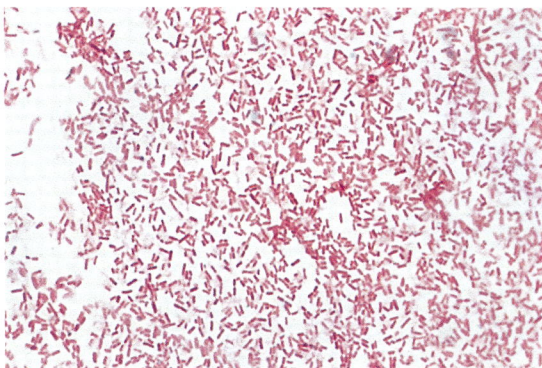

Fig. 6.1
Stool culture showing Gram-negative *Salmonella* organisms.

DIAGNOSIS
The onset of acute enteric symptoms in two people who shared the same meal is in keeping with an acute infective gastroenteritis. *Campylobacter jejuni* and *Salmonella enteritidis* are the commonest causes of bacterial gastroenteritis in the UK. Viral infections may produce a similar enteric illness. The incubation period of 24 h is consistent with salmonella infection (c.f. campylobacter infection in which the incubation period is 3–5 days). Most salmonella infections are contracted from foods such as eggs, dairy products and poultry that have either been poorly refrigerated or improperly cooked.

Most of the investigations are normal. Urea and electrolytes are usually normal because of the short duration of the symptoms and are seldom helpful in young healthy persons. Mild ketonuria, as seen in this case, is common in subjects who have been fasting or have been unable to eat because of illness.

OUTCOME
Miss McIntosh was rehydrated with intravenous saline. Her symptoms rapidly subsided and she was discharged 48 h after admission. The local public health physicians were notified of the diagnosis.

KEY POINTS

History/Examination
- Acute onset of vomiting with diarrhoea and abdominal pain is suggestive of an acute enteritis.
- The presence of a similar illness in a person who had shared the same meal is indicative of a common source of infection.

Investigations
- Stool cultures are important in diagnosis. Blood cultures can be helpful although they are negative in many cases.

Outcome
- In most cases of salmonellosis the symptoms are self-limiting and antibiotic therapy is not necessary.
- Salmonellosis is a notifiable infection in the UK.

Alexander Green (69)
Abdominal pain, collapse

CASE HISTORY
Mr Green, a retired driving instructor, had been troubled for a few weeks with intermittent central abdominal discomfort radiating through to his back. He attributed this to recent back strain caused by moving furniture, but when it started to wake him at night he arranged to see his general practitioner. On the morning of his appointment, he was suddenly overcome by a severe pain in the centre of his back radiating through to his upper abdomen. He was sweating profusely, felt nauseated and light-headed, and collapsed to the floor. An ambulance was called and he was admitted to hospital. Further enquiry revealed that he had suffered for some years from bilateral cramping pain in his calves when he walked, causing him to stop and rest every 100 m or so. More recently he had also been aware of central chest tightness when walking, particularly on cold or windy days.

Past medical history included sciatica 20 years ago, laryngoscopy 4 years ago for hoarseness (which showed only some chronic inflammation), and recurrent winter bronchitis. He drank around 10 units of alcohol per week, and smoked 30–40 cigarettes per day.

EXAMINATION
On admission, Mr Green was pale and sweating, distressed by his pain, and a little drowsy. He had tar-stained fingers. His pulse was 116/min and regular, and blood pressure was 92/66. The heart sounds were normal and there were no added sounds on auscultation of the lungs. There was some upper abdominal tenderness over a pulsatile central mass, but no organomegaly. There were bilateral carotid bruits and a left femoral bruit; the right femoral pulse was only weakly palpable and there were no detectable pulses in the feet. The only neurological deficit was absence of the right ankle jerk.

INVESTIGATIONS
Routine investigation results

Urine	SpG 1.014	Pr tr	Glu neg	Ke neg	Blood tr
Serum	Na 137	K 4.3	HCO_3 28	U 9.3	Cr 128
	Alb 38	Bil 20	AAT 26	AP 104	γGT 32
Blood	Hb 156	MCV 87	WCC 9.0	Plt 237	ESR 12

Additional investigations
Serum amylase was 326 U/l (reference range <340). An ECG showed sinus tachycardia with some lateral T-wave flattening. A chest radiograph showed unfolding and calcification of the aorta (Fig. 7.1). A lateral abdominal radiograph showed some further aortic calcification (Fig. 7.2). An abdominal ultrasound scan showed the presence of an aortic aneurysm (Fig. 7.3).

DIAGNOSIS
The history of angina and intermittent claudication indicated that this man had widespread arteriopathy. His increasing abdominal/back pain with sudden exacerbation and collapse therefore suggested the presence of an aortic aneurysm which had dissected and was perhaps leaking. The clinical picture of shock with a pulsatile central abdominal swelling supported this diagnosis, and the inequality of the femoral pulses was also consistent with aortic dissection. The

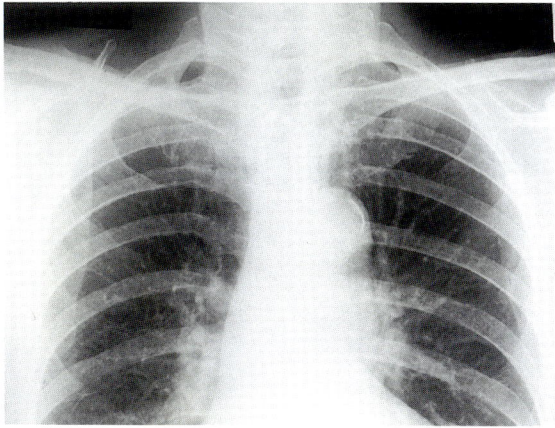

Fig. 7.1
Chest radiograph showing unfolded, calcified aorta.

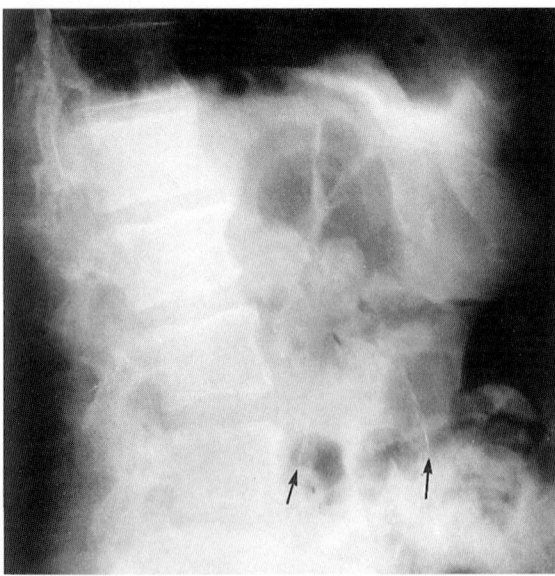

Fig. 7.2
Lateral abdominal radiograph showing calcification in an aneurysmal aorta (arrows).

abdominal ultrasound scan quickly confirmed the suspected diagnosis, demonstrating the aneurysmal swelling of the aorta. The ECG did not show features of acute myocardial infarction. The absent ankle jerk was unrelated to his current problem, and was probably the result of lumbar nerve root compression which had given rise to his previous complaint of sciatica. Catheterization was necessary to monitor urine output (and to obtain a urine specimen), and the trace of haematuria noted was therefore to be expected and of no pathological significance.

OUTCOME

The patient was treated with analgesia and careful use of plasma expander to partially restore his blood pressure before emergency aorto-bifemoral grafting. The operation was uneventful but the postoperative course was complicated by acute renal failure (acute tubular necrosis due to the hypotensive episode) and lateral myocardial infarction. This illustrated how disease of the cardiovascular system may manifest itself in a number of ways in a given patient, and how patients with severe cardiovascular disease are particularly susceptible to the complications of a hypotensive episode. Mr Green eventually made a reasonable recovery and was discharged home 6 weeks after admission. Unfortunately, he quickly resumed his smoking habits.

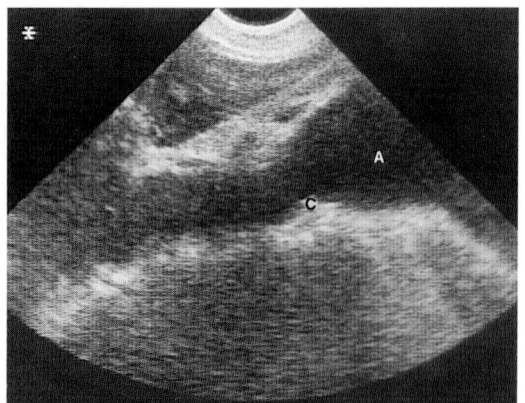
(a)

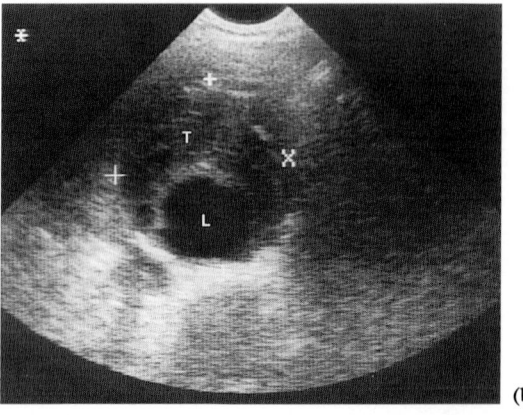
(b)

Fig. 7.3
(a) Longitudinal abdominal ultrasound scan image showing aneurysmal dilatation of the aorta (A) with calcification in the vessel wall (C). (b) Transverse abdominal ultrasound scan image showing aortic aneurysm, intraluminal thrombus (T) and residual lumen (L). Caliper crosses indicate maximum aortic diameter of 7.5 cm.

KEY POINTS

History/Examination
- Smoking is the most important single risk factor for cardiovascular diseases.
- Consider aortic disease as a cause of back/abdominal pain.
- Unequal femoral pulses can be due to aortic dissection.

Investigations
- Remember to look for aortic calcification on abdominal radiographs.
- Ultrasound scanning is a simple, non-invasive means of assessing the abdominal aorta.

Outcome
- A patient with an aortic dissection or aneurysmal leak can make an excellent recovery if resuscitation and surgical repair are carried out promptly.

James Wright (68) Haematemesis

CASE HISTORY

Mr Wright had complained of feeling nauseated following lunch. About 5 h later, he felt faint and 'blacked out' for about 3 min. His wife said that during this episode he looked pale, but he had no twitching or incontinence and did not injure himself. Following recovery he called his general practitioner, on whose arrival he vomited a substantial volume of bright red blood and again felt faint. He had recently been complaining of slight indigestion relieved by eating but had no other specific complaints and, in particular, had not noticed any change in bowel habit or dark stools.

He had a previous history of alcohol abuse at the age of 55 years and had been abstinent for the past 8 years. He had suffered angina since the age of 64 years, and had a transient cerebral ischaemic attack 2 years prior to his current illness. He had no previous history of peptic ulceration and there was no family history of ulcer disease. He had suffered a painful right hip since 60 years of age, and a recent radiograph of the pelvis had revealed osteoarthritis of the hip joint (Fig. 8.1). He was an ex-smoker, having stopped 5 years previously, and lived with his wife in a ground floor flat. He was taking a calcium antagonist and a long-acting nitrate for angina prophylaxis, a non-steroidal anti-inflammatory drug (NSAID) and aspirin (150 mg/day).

EXAMINATION

He was pale, sweaty and anxious. His pulse was 120/min, regular with occasional missed beats, and blood pressure was 100/70. The heart sounds were normal and there was no evidence of cardiac failure. The respiratory system was normal. There were no palpable abdominal masses, but he was slightly tender in the epigastrium and the bowel sounds were active. Rectal examination was normal but the faecal occult blood test was positive. Neurological examination was normal. There was limitation of flexion and rotation of his right hip due to pain.

INVESTIGATIONS

Routine investigation results

Urine	SpG 1020	Pr neg	Glu neg	Ke neg	Blood neg
Serum	Na 138	K 4.3	HCO_3 27	U 14.5	Cr 88
	Alb 44	Bil 8	AAT 12	AP 63	γGT 24
Blood	Hb 108	MCV 79	WCC 9.4	Plt 228	ESR 18

Additional investigations

Upper gastrointestinal endoscopy showed fresh and altered blood in the stomach and duodenum. There was no evidence of oesophageal varices, but scattered superficial erosions were seen (Fig. 8.2), some of which were actively bleeding at the time of endoscopy.

DIAGNOSIS

The diagnosis is gastrointestinal haemorrhage due to gastric erosions. These are secondary to the use of aspirin and an NSAID. Endoscopy was important in this case to specify the cause of the haemorrhage and to exclude the presence of a peptic ulcer or oesophageal or gastric varices in view of the previous history of alcohol excess.

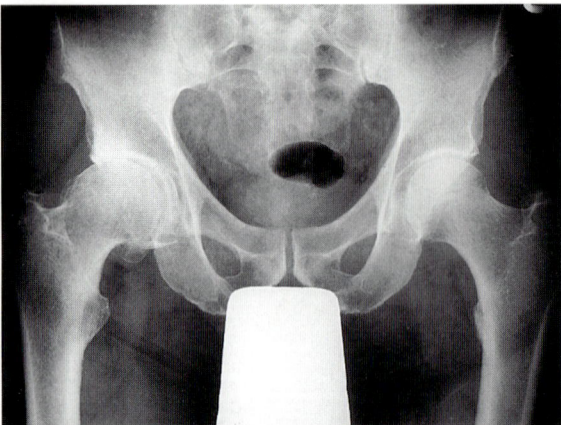

Fig. 8.1
Antero-posterior radiograph of both hips showing osteoarthritis of the right hip with loss of superior joint space and subchondral sclerosis.

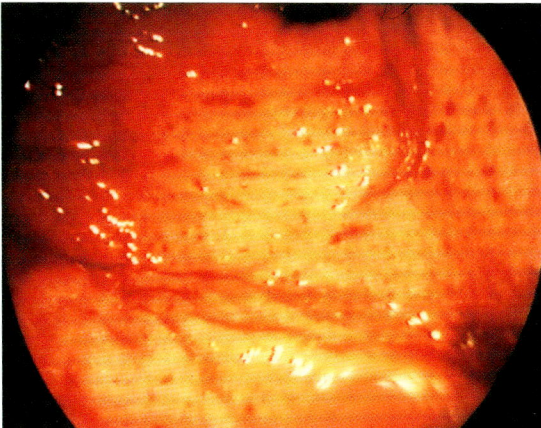

Fig. 8.2
Endoscopic view of the gastric mucosa showing multiple haemorrhagic erosions.

The haemoglobin level is often normal immediately after an acute haemorrhage and falls later as haemodilution occurs. Elevation of the blood urea, a normal creatinine and the presence of active bowel sounds suggest that substantial acute blood loss into the gastrointestinal tract has occurred. The reduced haemoglobin and MCV at presentation suggest that, in addition to the acute haemorrhage, there has been chronic blood loss.

OUTCOME
Mr Wright was treated with intravenous fluids, transfusion of 3 units of packed red cells and intravenous and subsequent oral H_2-receptor blocking agents. The aspirin and NSAID were stopped, and he was advised to use paracetamol for the pain in his hip. He made an uncomplicated recovery.

KEY POINTS
History/Examination
- Aspirin and other NSAIDs may cause acute gastric erosions.
- Tachycardia, hypotension and the presence of active bowel sounds suggest that a significant gastrointestinal haemorrhage has occurred.

Investigations
- The haemoglobin level is a poor indicator of the degree of an acute haemorrhage and may be normal in the presence of a life-threatening haemorrhage.

Outcome
- Close monitoring of the haemodynamic state of the patient is essential in cases of gastrointestinal haemorrhage.
- Aspirin and other NSAIDs should be avoided in patients with a history of peptic ulcer symptoms.

George Speed (68)
Breathlessness, weight loss

CASE HISTORY
Mr Speed, a retired railway guard, was referred urgently to the medical outpatient clinic with increasing breathlessness on exertion and tiredness over the previous 2 months. He had a poor appetite and thought he had lost a lot of weight. He had had a dry cough for a month, and a week before referral had coughed up some red-brown streaked sputum. His legs had been weak and he had a dull pain around his wrists and ankles.

Previous medical history included inguinal herniorrhaphy and hypertension, for which he was taking a calcium-channel blocking drug. There was no family history of note; Mr Speed's wife was in poor health following a stroke the previous year. He smoked 20 cigarettes per day and drank little alcohol. As a result of his presenting features he was admitted directly to hospital for investigation.

EXAMINATION
He appeared pale and underweight. He had tar-stained nails and finger clubbing. There was slight tenderness over his forearms, wrists and ankles. There was no lymphadenopathy. He was tachypnoeic on even minor exertion. His resting pulse was 90/min, and blood pressure was 140/95. The trachea was central and the thyroid gland impalpable. There was lower, anterior, right-sided dullness on percussion and reduced breath sounds in the same area. Heart sounds were normal. Posteriorly, examination of the chest, including expansion, was normal. There were no abdominal masses or hepatic enlargement. Despite his complaint of weakness there was no abnormality on formal neurological examination.

INVESTIGATIONS
Routine investigation results

Urine	SpG 1.030	Pr neg	Glu neg	Ke neg	Blood neg
Serum	Na 135	K 3.6	HCO_3 29	U 8.5	Cr 122
	Alb 30	Bil 5	AAT 12	AP 69	γGT 34
Blood	Hb 125	MCV 83	WCC 8.1	Plt 387	ESR 64

Additional investigations
Random blood glucose was 7.4 mmol/l (reference range <8.0), serum calcium 2.02 mmol/l (2.20–2.60), serum thyroxine 72 nmol/l (70–150) and TSH 1.7 mU/l (0.35–3.30). Sputum culture was negative; microscopy showed no mycobacteria. Sputum cytology showed atypical, possibly malignant, cells on one of three specimens, but a definite diagnosis was not possible.

An ECG showed sinus rhythm and no abnormal features. Postero-anterior and right lateral chest radiographs (Fig. 9.1) were abnormal. Radiography of the wrists showed periosteal abnormality (Fig. 9.2). CT showed a mass at the lower pole of the right hilum associated with right middle lobe consolidation and involvement of the adjacent mediastinum (Fig. 9.3). At bronchoscopy, tumour tissue was seen at the origin of the middle lobe bronchus. Biopsy and brushings were taken, which showed large cell anaplastic carcinoma.

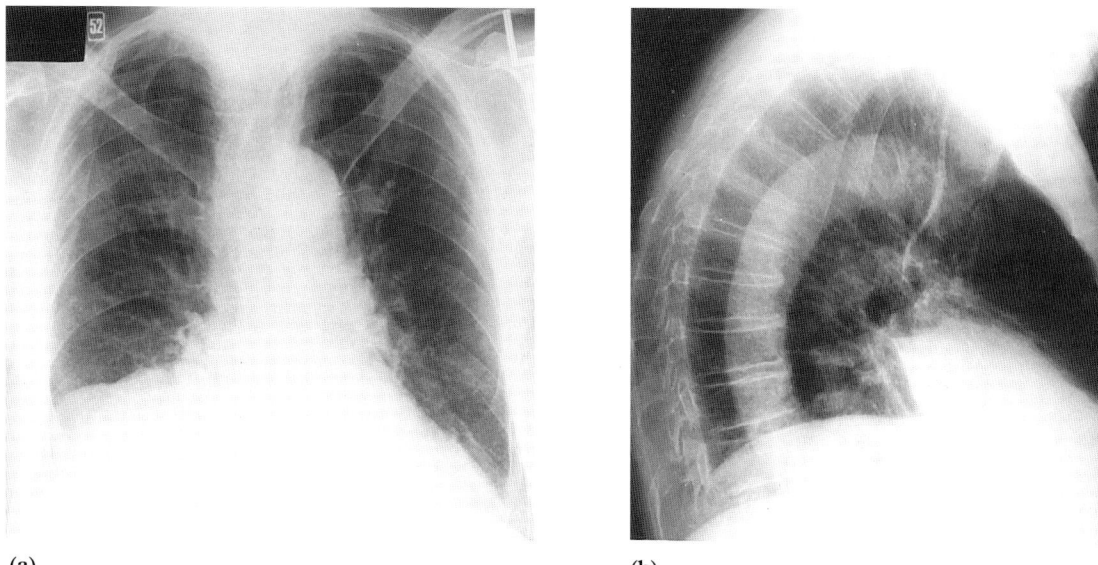

(a) (b)

Fig. 9.1
(a) Postero-anterior chest radiograph showing right lower zone opacification. (b) Right lateral chest radiograph showing opacification situated anteriorly, in the middle lobe.

DIAGNOSIS

This man had an inoperable carcinoma of the bronchus causing non-specific systemic features including weight loss, anorexia and lethargy, and contributing to his exertional dyspnoea by reducing the volume of functioning lung tissue. The history of weight loss and malaise suggested an underlying malignant process, although other causes such as tuberculosis and hyperthyroidism also had to be considered; haemoptysis made bronchial carcinoma or tuberculosis the most likely diagnoses. The history of smoking and the presence of finger clubbing (which is often absent) were important diagnostic clues. The probable diagnosis was only proven by histological examination of the specimens obtained at bronchoscopy. The normocytic anaemia, high ESR and low serum albumin are all non-specific features of

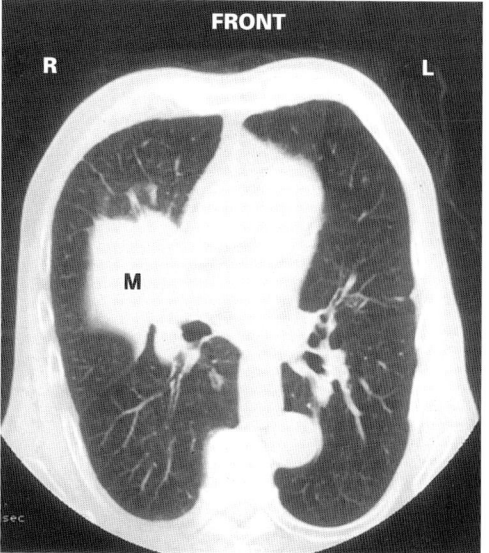

Fig. 9.2
Radiograph of the wrist showing the periosteal thickening (arrow) of hypertrophic pulmonary osteoarthropathy.

Fig. 9.3
Single transverse CT section through the chest at the level of the hila showing a right lower pole hilar mass (M).

systemic illness. The serum calcium was low on account of the low serum albumin concentration, and physiologically active (ionized) calcium would be expected to be normal; the 'corrected' serum calcium was normal at 2.27 mmol/l (calculated by adding 0.025 mmol per gram of albumin under 40 g/l). The discomfort in his wrists and ankles was due to hypertrophic pulmonary osteoarthropathy, which is an occasional non-metastatic complication of bronchial carcinoma.

There was no evidence of metastatic disease in this patient although this is often in evidence at presentation.

OUTCOME
The tumour was unresectable due to invasion into the mediastinum as shown by the CT scan. Mr Speed underwent a course of palliative radiotherapy which he tolerated well. His general condition improved a little and he managed to spend 3 months at home with his wife before there was a secondary deterioration and he developed a bronchopneumonia and died.

KEY POINTS

History/Examination
- Involuntary weight loss and malaise are suggestive of malignant disease, particularly in the middle-aged and elderly.
- A smoker with haemoptysis should be regarded as having bronchial carcinoma until proven otherwise.
- Chest signs may be relatively unremarkable in the presence of advanced pulmonary malignancy.

Investigations
- Sputum cytology is helpful when positive, but is often negative in the presence of bronchial carcinoma.
- Histological specimens of central pulmonary lesions are best obtained by bronchoscopic procedures.
- CT scanning is of particular use in the assessment of operability of bronchial carcinoma.

Outcome
- Most bronchial carcinomas are unsuitable for resection at presentation, due either to local invasion or detectable metastatic disease.

Mary Stanley (66) Chest pain

CASE HISTORY
Mrs Stanley, a housewife, woke up at 4 am with severe central chest tightness radiating to the throat. The pain gradually eased over the next hour, allowing her to go back to sleep, but 3h later, while having breakfast, she had further chest pain. On this occasion it was more severe and associated with nausea, vomiting and sweating. Her general practitioner gave her an analgesic injection at home and 45 min later she arrived in hospital.

She had previously suffered chest tightness when shopping or walking uphill. Her general practitioner had diagnosed angina and had prescribed sublingual glyceryl trinitrate, which she took once or twice per week to relieve her symptoms. She took no other regular medication. Her younger brother had died 4 years previously of a 'heart attack'. She was married with two children and had smoked 20 cigarettes daily for 30 years. She had been diabetic since the age of 50 years and this was controlled by diet.

EXAMINATION
On admission she was drowsy and obese but there was no fever, cyanosis or pallor. Her pulse was 87/min, regular and of good volume, and blood pressure was 120/70. Auscultation of the praecordium and respiratory examination were normal, as were abdominal and nervous system examination. Fundoscopy showed evidence of diabetic retinopathy (Fig. 10.1).

INVESTIGATIONS
Routine investigation results

Urine	SpG 1.010	Pr neg	Glu +	Ke neg	Blood neg
Serum	Na 140	K 4.0	HCO₃ 24	U 5.6	Cr 98
	Alb 35	Bil 13	AAT 41	AP 50	γGT 35
Blood	Hb 127	MCV 92	WCC 9.8	Plt 242	ESR 17

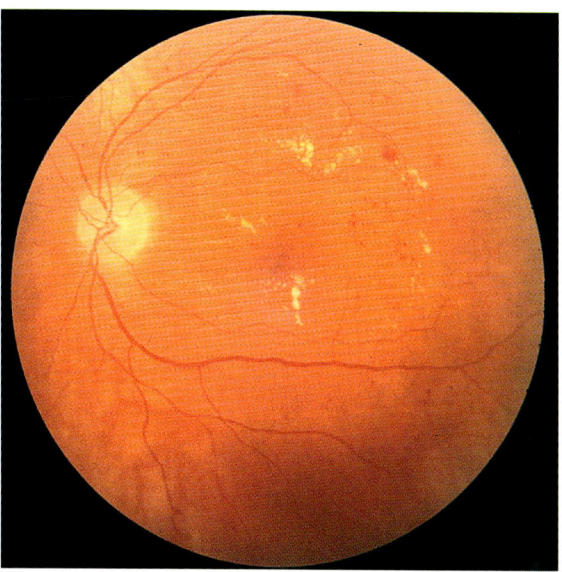

Fig. 10.1
Fundoscopic view showing dot and blot haemorrhages and hard exudates typical of diabetic background retinopathy.

Additional investigations
Creatine kinase (CK) was 800 U/l (reference range <50) and CK-MB isoenzyme was elevated (70% of total CK). Serum lactate dehydrogenase (LDH) was 345 U/l (reference range <250). An ECG (Fig. 10.2) on admission was abnormal. Serum cholesterol was 7 mmol/l (reference range <5.2), and random blood glucose was 13.3 mmol/l (reference range <8).

DIAGNOSIS
The history of prolonged gripping central chest pain, radiating to the neck, associated with vomiting and sweating is highly suggestive of an acute myocardial infarction, although alternative causes such as oesophageal spasm, pericarditis, pulmonary embolism and aortic dissection should be considered. The fact that she is a smoker and is diabetic with a previous history of angina adds to the probability of myocardial ischaemia as a cause for her symptoms. The diagnosis of acute inferior myocardial infarction is confirmed by the elevated cardiac enzymes and ECG abnormalities apparent in the inferior leads (leads II, III and aVF).

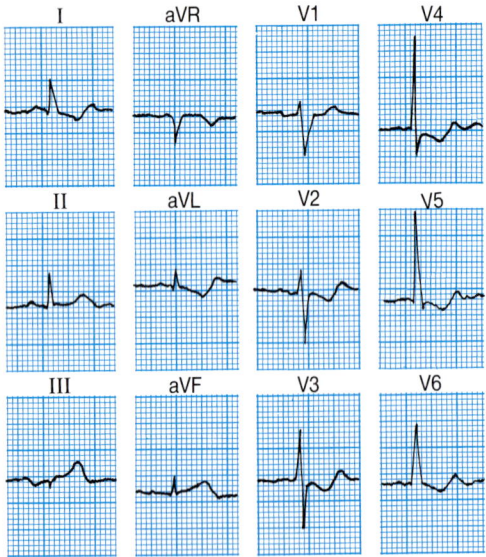

Fig. 10.2
ECG on admission showing slight ST elevation in leads II, III and aVF with reciprocal ST depression in I, aVL and V2–V6.

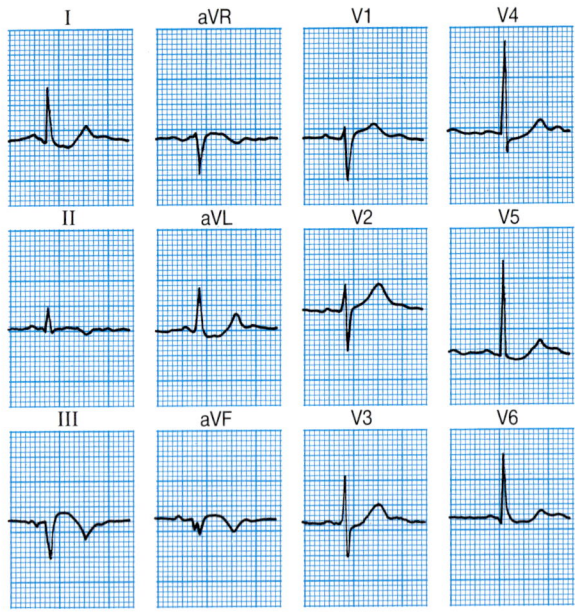

Fig. 10.3
ECG 3 days after admission showing Q waves in leads III and aVF with T-wave inversion in leads II, III and aVF.

The most specific cardiac enzyme available is an isoenzyme of creatine kinase (CK) called the MB fraction (CK-MB). The level rises within hours of the infarction and falls within 24–48 h. Aspartate aminotransferase is usually raised 24–48 h after infarction. It is non-specific and, for example, is also elevated in damage to liver or lung tissue. Lactate dehydrogenase (LDH) appears in the blood within 12–24 h after infarction and may remain elevated for some days. The most characteristic feature of infarction on the 12-lead ECG is the development of ST segment elevation with a convex upward pattern in the leads facing the area of ventricle infarcted. Later changes of infarction, seen in this case, include the appearance of Q waves and T wave inversion (Fig. 10.3).

OUTCOME
Mrs Stanley was given intravenous diamorphine, an antiemetic and thrombolytic therapy with intravenous streptokinase. She was commenced on oral aspirin.

She made an uneventful recovery and was discharged home 6 days later. She was advised to stop smoking and given further dietary advice. Arrangements were made for review in 6 weeks to consider further investigations such as exercise stress testing.

KEY POINTS

History/Examination
- Gripping central chest pain radiating to the neck, associated with vomiting and sweating, is typical of acute myocardial infarction.
- Smoking, obesity, hypertension, diabetes, hyperlipidaemia and a family history of ischaemic heart disease are important risk factors for myocardial infarction.

Investigations
- Serial measurements of cardiac enzymes and electrocardiography are used to diagnose myocardial infarction.

Outcome
- Thrombolytic therapy reduces infarct size and acute mortality from myocardial infarction.

Frederick James (70) Breathlessness, anaemia

CASE HISTORY
Mr James, a 70-year-old retired executive, attended his general practitioner for an annual assessment of his blood pressure. He mentioned that he had noticed breathlessness on exertion such as playing the steeper holes on his local golf course. For the past 6 months he had also been feeling rather lethargic. He denied any other symptoms but the general practitioner noted that he looked rather pale, and on checking his blood count, found him to be anaemic and referred him to hospital for investigation. On further questioning, he again denied any other symptoms. His appetite was normal and his weight was steady. He had not noticed any change in the colour of his stools nor had he seen blood in the stools.

He had a previous history of pneumonia aged 65 years. He was a lifelong non-smoker and drank six units of alcohol per week. There was no family history of anaemia or blood disorders. He was not taking medication.

EXAMINATION
He was a fit-looking man but had marked pallor of the mucous membranes. He had deformed nails (Fig. 11.1), but general examination was otherwise negative. His pulse was 100/min, regular and blood pressure was 150/90. Heart sounds were normal and there was a soft systolic murmur audible in the aortic area with no radiation to the neck. The respiratory system was normal and abdominal examination was negative. Rectal examination was normal but the faecal occult blood test was positive. There was no neurological abnormality.

INVESTIGATIONS
Routine investigation results

Urine	SpG 1005	Pr neg	Glu neg	Ke neg	Blood neg
Serum	Na 139	K 4.5	HCO₃ 24	U 3.3	Cr 90
	Alb 38	Bil 13	AAT 17	AP 90	γGT 24
Blood	Hb 66	MCV 60	WCC 6.6	Plt 553	ESR 36

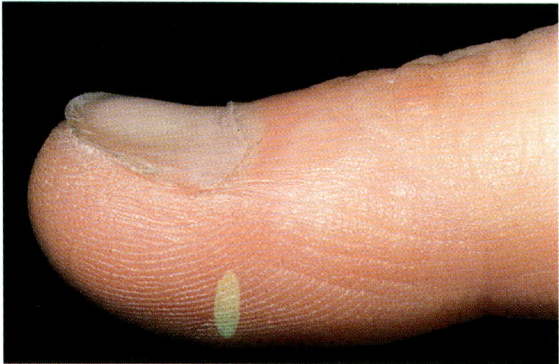

Fig. 11.1
Appearances of the finger nail (koilonychia).

Additional investigations
Serum iron was 10 μmol/l (reference range 13–32) and serum ferritin was 5.2 μg/l (20–350). Sigmoidoscopy was normal, but a barium enema (Fig. 11.2) was abnormal. An abdominal ultrasound scan showed no masses and normal appearances of liver and spleen.

DIAGNOSIS
He was anaemic, and the low MCV, serum iron and ferritin confirmed this was iron deficiency anaemia, which proved to be secondary to blood loss from a carcinoma of the ascending colon. Tumours of the caecum and ascending colon often present with anaemia alone. Intestinal obstruction or local invasion or metastasis of these tumours tend to occur late. In contrast, intestinal obstruction may be an early presenting feature of tumours in the descending and sigmoid colon. The presence of koilonychia suggests that the anaemia has been present for months.

The cardiac murmur is a flow murmur related to the increased cardiac output associated with anaemia. Flow murmurs, which arise from a normal heart, may be heard in other situations in which cardiac output is increased, e.g. pregnancy, thyrotoxicosis.

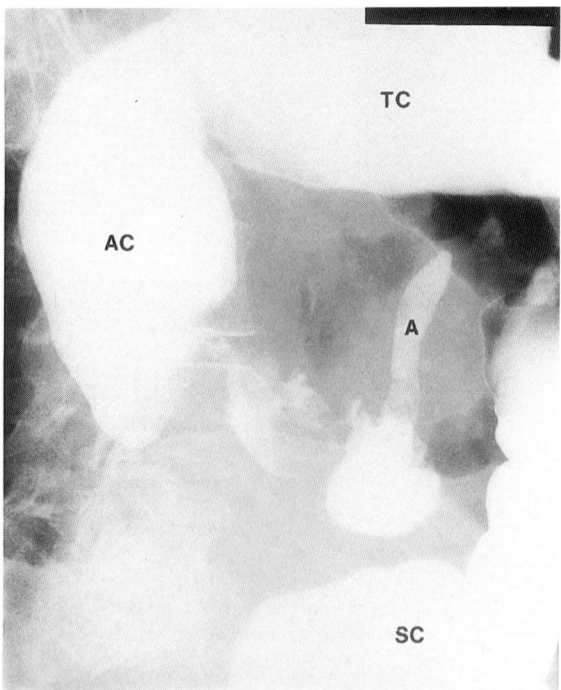

Fig. 11.2
Double-contrast barium enema showing a concentric stricturing of the caecum with mucosal destruction and everted edges (apple core lesion): AC, ascending colon; TC, transverse colon; SC, sigmoid colon; A, appendix.

OUTCOME

Mr James received a tranfusion of four units of packed red blood cells before proceeding to laparotomy, which confirmed the presence of a carcinoma of the caecum. There was no evidence of metastatic disease. Right hemicolectomy was performed and the ileum was anastomosed directly to the transverse colon. Histologically the tumour had not penetrated the thickness of the bowel wall and the lymph nodes were negative.

He made an uncomplicated recovery from surgery and was given a 1-month course of oral iron supplements. At review 2 months later he was well, and the cardiac murmur was no longer present.

KEY POINTS

History/Examination
- Significant gastrointestinal blood loss may occur without it being observed by the patient.
- Clinical examination of the abdomen may be normal even when serious abdominal pathology is present.

Investigations
- Barium enema is an essential investigation in a patient with anaemia and evidence of gastrointestinal blood loss of unknown cause.

Outcome
- Curative surgery for colonic carcinoma is more feasible after early diagnosis.

Paul Reeves (17)
Sore throat, rash

CASE HISTORY

Mr Reeves was admitted to hospital complaining of a sore throat, pain on swallowing and fever. Two days before admission he had seen his general practitioner who had prescribed amoxycillin for a suspected bacterial throat infection. Shortly after starting the antibiotic, he had developed a rash. Apart from his sore throat he also complained of 'lack of energy' and had noticed a dull ache under his left rib margin.

His previous health had been good. He was a non-smoker and lived with his parents. He had recently started college.

EXAMINATION

He was miserable, febrile and dehydrated. He had a macular rash over his arms, abdomen and legs (Fig. 12.1) and had marked bilateral cervical and axillary lymphadenopathy. Examination of the mouth showed white exudates over oedematous fauces (Fig. 12.2) and palatal petechiae (Fig. 12.3). There was a smooth, non-tender, palpable liver edge 2 cm below the costal margin and a moderately enlarged tender spleen. The remainder of the examination was normal.

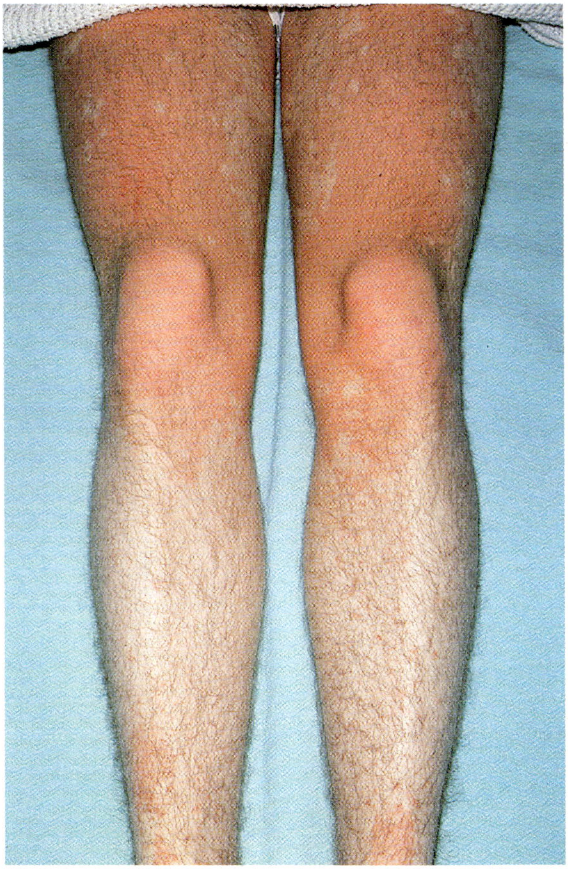

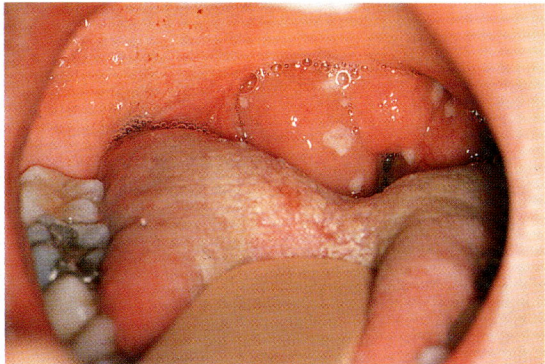

Fig. 12.2
Oedematous fauces with patchy exudate.

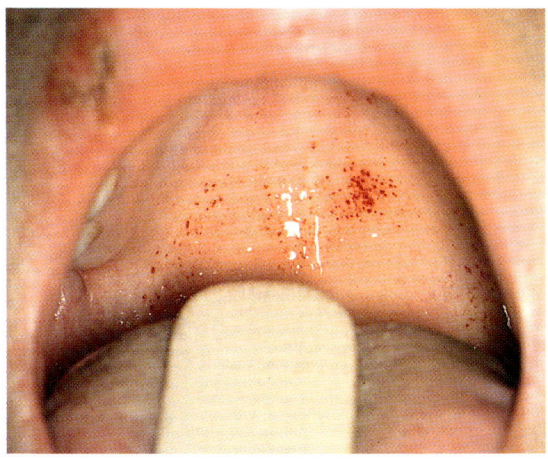

Fig. 12.1
Macular rash, typical of drug eruption.

Fig. 12.3
Palatal petechiae.

INVESTIGATIONS
Routine investigation results

Urine	SpG 1.021	Pr neg	Glu neg	Ke neg	Blood neg
Serum	Na 139	K 3.9	HCO$_3$ 28	U 6.9	Cr 101
	Alb 44	Bil 35	AAT 89	AP 268	γGT 70
Blood	Hb 120	MCV 90	WCC 4.5	Plt 378	ESR 89

Additional investigations
A differential white cell count showed 70% lymphocytes, 18% monocytes and 3% neutrophils. The blood film showed scanty atypical mononuclear cells. An infectious mononucleosis spot test (Monospot) was positive. Throat and blood bacterial cultures were negative. The serum antistreptolysin O titre (ASO) was <160; Epstein Barr virus (EBV)-specific IgM was positive.

DIAGNOSIS
The association of fever, lymphadenopathy, sore throat and systemic upset with a peripheral blood monocytosis in a young adult is very suggestive of infectious mononucleosis (glandular fever). The diagnosis is confirmed by the positive (Monospot) test. The occurrence of a rash after taking a semisynthetic penicillin and biochemical evidence of hepatitis are very common in infectious mononucleosis, as seen in this case. The disease is caused by EBV; EBV-specific IgM antibody appears and disappears early in the course of the illness.

Cytomegalovirus, toxoplasmosis and HIV infection, amongst others, can produce a similar syndrome but are differentiated by a negative Monospot. When throat symptoms and signs predominate, differentiation from streptococcal tonsillitis has to be made. A negative throat swab and normal ASO titre will exclude the latter diagnosis.

Complications of IM are uncommon but include splenic rupture, frank jaundice, thrombocytopenia with purpura and bleeding, and meningitis or encephalitis.

OUTCOME
Mr Reeves was treated symptomatically with intravenous fluids and analgesia. He showed considerable improvement over the next few days. The rash subsided and the fever settled on no antibiotics. He was discharged on no medication.

KEY POINTS

History/Examination
- Glandular fever should be suspected in a young person who is systemically unwell with a sore throat.
- The macular rash (Fig. 12.1) is typical of a drug eruption.

Investigations
- Atypical lymphocytes on the blood film are suggestive of infectious mononucleosis.
- The Monospot test allows rapid diagnosis, but may be negative in the early stages of infection and may have to be repeated.

Outcome
- Symptomatic treatment only is necessary in most cases.

Thomas Wildgoose (67)
Chest infection, drowsiness

CASE HISTORY
Mr Wildgoose, a retired bus driver, was unwell and in bed with a cough and general malaise when he called in his general practitioner. An upper respiratory tract infection was diagnosed and erythromycin prescribed. Two days later, at a second home visit, he was found to be a little breathless and complaining that he felt worse. He was advised to drink plenty and to continue with his antibiotic. Another 2 days passed and the general practitioner returned to find the patient barely rousable and breathless at rest. Emergency admission to hospital was arranged on the grounds of 'severe chest infection'. On arrival in the ward, he was unable to give any history but it was ascertained from his wife that he had been confused and unable to get up for the previous 24h. He had been incontinent of urine on a few occasions during this time. He had been noted to have increased thirst and nocturia for the previous 2 weeks.

His past history included appendicectomy at age 11 years, cervical spondylosis 10 years ago, and hypertension for which he had been taking a thiazide diuretic for 3 years. His father had died at 62 years of myocardial infarction and his mother had had rheumatoid arthritis. His wife kept generally well but had also had a throat infection the previous week. Mr Wildgoose drank little alcohol and had stopped smoking 2 years previously.

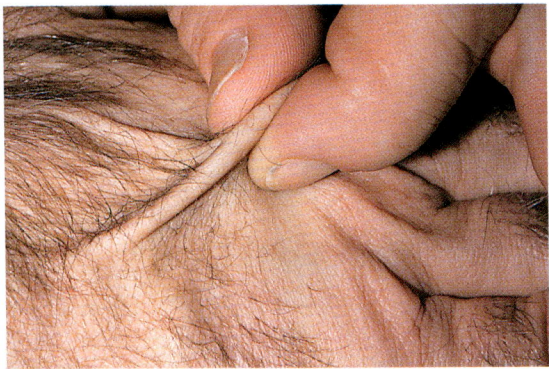

Fig. 13.1 Reduced skin turgor indicating marked dehydration.

EXAMINATION
The patient was overweight, restless and tachypnoeic. He was semiconscious and confused. He was apyrexial and in fact had cool extremities and some peripheral cyanosis. His tongue and lips were dry and he had reduced skin turgor (Fig. 13.1). His fauces were reddened. His pulse was 110/min and regular, and blood pressure was 100/56. The jugular venous pulse was not visible. There were no abnormal findings in the chest. The abdomen was soft and non-tender with no organomegaly, and bowel sounds were present. There was no neck stiffness to indicate meningism and there were no focal neurological signs. Plantar responses were flexor and fundi normal.

INVESTIGATIONS
Routine investigation results

Urine	SpG 1.028	Pr tr	Glu ++++	Ke neg	Blood neg
Serum	Na 150	K 5.9	HCO_3 13	U 35.4	Cr 338
	Alb 31	Bil 15	AAT 68	AP 111	γGT 32
Blood	Hb 168	MCV 91	WCC 15.0	Plt 314	ESR 59

Additional investigations
Blood glucose was 58.1 mmol/l (reference range <8.0) and arterial blood gases were as follows:

pH	pO_2	pCO_2	$sHCO_3$
7.28	8.9	3.1	15

Blood lactate 8.6 mmol/l (0–2). An ECG showed sinus tachycardia and features of left ventricular hypertrophy (Fig. 13.2). A chest radiograph (Fig. 13.3) showed clear lung fields and cardiac enlargement. There was no growth from blood cultures and a throat swab showed normal oral flora; no pathogens were isolated.

DIAGNOSIS
This man was severely ill due to a hyperosmolar non-ketotic diabetic state, as evidenced by marked hyperglycaemia in the absence of ketonuria. Serum

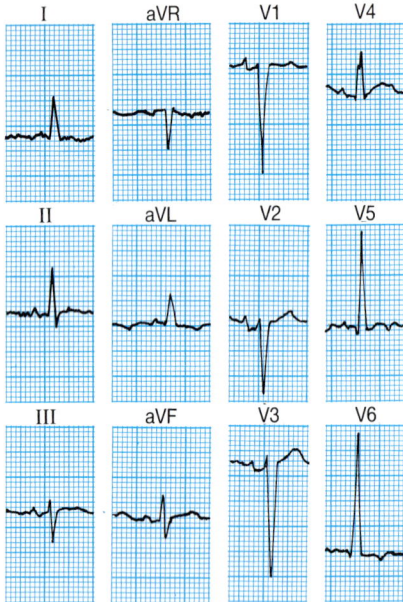

Fig. 13.2
ECG complexes showing features of left ventricular hypertrophy.

osmolality was greatly elevated at approximately 405 mOsm/kg (calculated from the formula 2 × [Na + K] + urea + glucose). Tissue perfusion was poor owing to the combination of acidosis and dehydration leading to the peripheral cyanosis, and tissue hypoxia had led to lactic acidosis. The elevation in urea and creatinine was also due to dehydration with reduced renal blood flow ('pre-renal' uraemia). The precipitating event was probably the physiological stress of an acute upper respiratory infection, aggravated by his thiazide therapy and increased consumption of sweetened drinks in an attempt to quench his thirst.

There was no clinical or radiological evidence of the chest infection that had been suspected on the basis of tachypnoea in an obviously unwell patient. His hyperventilation, as he attempted to correct a metabolic acidosis by blowing off increased amounts of carbon dioxide, had been mistaken for a primary respiratory problem. In this case, the acidosis was predominantly due to an accumulation of lactate, a common consequence of tissue hypoperfusion of various aetiologies.

Left ventricular hypertrophy was considered to be present on the ECG as the combined 'heights' of the S wave in lead V1, and R wave in lead V5 exceeded 35 mm; cardiac enlargement was said to be present on the postero-anterior chest radiograph as the maximum transverse cardiac diameter exceeded 50% of the maximum transverse thoracic diameter ('increased cardiothoracic ratio'). The ECG and chest radiograph findings were both in keeping with sustained hypertension, and the blood pressure on admission (100/56) was therefore likely to be much lower than the usual levels for this patient.

OUTCOME

Treatment was commenced immediately with insulin infusion and cautious fluid and electrolyte replacement. Despite the significant mortality of this condition, Mr Wildgoose made an excellent recovery and was discharged home two and a half weeks later on a sugar-free, weight-reducing diet which had produced a random blood glucose of 8 mmol/l.

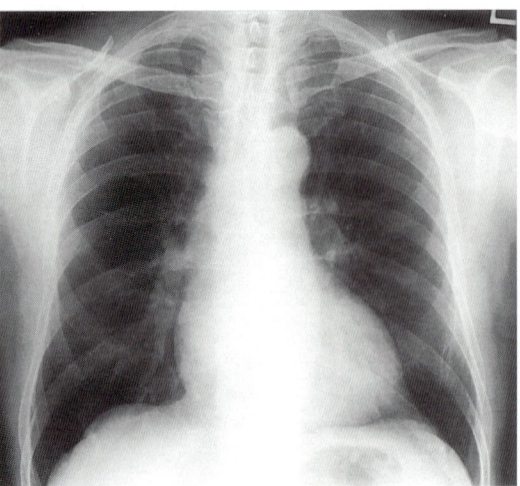

Fig. 13.3
Chest radiograph showing normal lung fields and increased cardiothoracic ratio.

KEY POINTS

History/Examination
- Consider hyperglycaemia in any unwell patient with a history of thirst and polyuria.
- Metabolic acidosis should be sought as a cause of apparent breathlessness in a patient without central cyanosis or abnormal chest signs.

Investigations
- Serum osmolality can be estimated from Na, K, urea and glucose concentrations.
- Acidosis in diabetes is not always due to ketosis.

Outcome
- Hyperosmolar, non-ketotic diabetic coma has a significant mortality.
- While insulin is required in the acute stages, normal blood glucose can be subsequently maintained by dietary measures alone in many cases.

William Stoddard (69) Dysphagia

CASE HISTORY
Mr Stoddard, a retired plumber, complained that for the past month he had been having increasing difficulty with swallowing. His wife had gradually modified his diet, initially cutting out meat and high fibre foods, and subsequently liquidizing much of his food. He had regurgitated virtually unaltered food on a number of occasions. During the last 24h, he had been able to swallow only liquids. He had lost about 12k in weight, and for about 2 weeks had noticed continuous dull aching lower chest pain.

He had a previous history of ischaemic heart disease, and was taking a calcium antagonist to prevent angina. He had undergone an appendicectomy at age 23 years and a lumbar laminectomy at age 35 years, but had had no other serious illnesses. He smoked 30 cigarettes daily and drank a few pints of beer each week.

EXAMINATION
He was thin and his general appearance suggested recent weight loss (Fig. 14.1). He had no lymphadenopathy or finger clubbing. His pulse was 96/min, and regular, and blood pressure was 130/90; heart sounds were normal. He had mild bilateral ankle oedema. His chest was hyperinflated and breath sounds were vesicular with prolonged expiration and some expiratory rhonchi. His abdomen was soft and non-tender. There was a scar from his previous appendicectomy but there were no palpable masses and bowel sounds were present. Rectal examination was normal but the faecal occult blood test was weakly positive. There were no focal neurological abnormalities.

INVESTIGATIONS
Routine investigation results

Urine	SpG 1015	Pr neg	Glu neg	Ke ++	Blood neg
Serum	Na 143	K 4.9	HCO$_3$ 24	U 11.6	Cr 124
	Alb 27	Bil 9	AAT 32	AP 107	γGT 31
Blood	Hb 124	MCV 78	WCC 9.3	Plt 380	ESR 38

Additional investigations
His chest radiograph was normal and the absence of a gastric air bubble was noted (Fig. 14.2). Barium swallow was abnormal (Fig. 14.3). The diagnosis was confirmed at oesophagosopy.

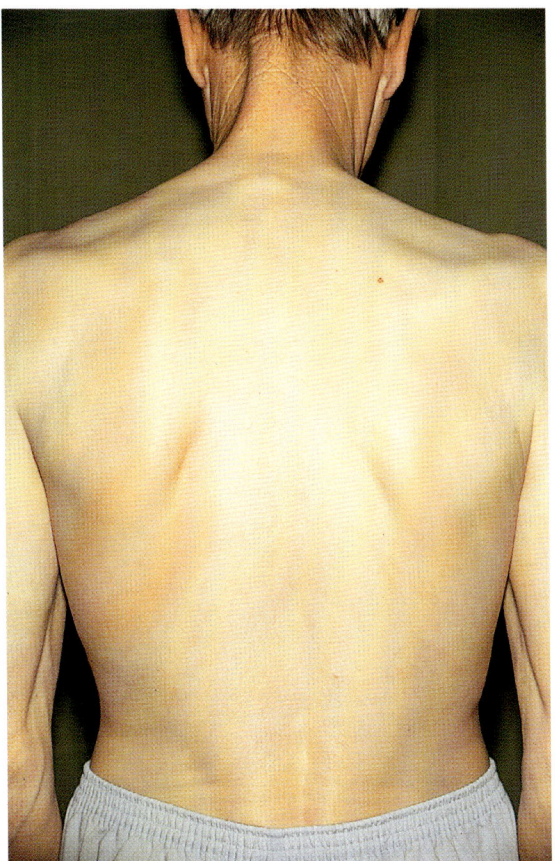

Fig. 14.1
Posterior view of the patient indicating weight loss. Note the scar from previous spinal surgery.

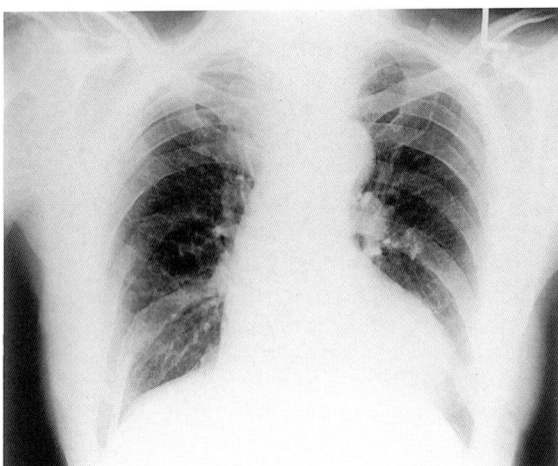

Fig. 14.2
Chest radiograph showing absence of gastric bubble.

DIAGNOSIS

The short history of rapidly progressive dysphagia and weight loss suggest that the likely diagnosis is oesophageal carcinoma. This was supported by the barium swallow, which showed almost complete occlusion of the lower end of the oesophagus by an irregular mass (Fig. 14.3). At oesophagoscopy, the mass was visualized at 28 cm from the lips and biopsies showed squamous carcinoma. A thoracic CT scan showed that the mass extended into the tissues of the lower mediastinum.

Oesophageal carcinoma is commoner in men than women, and there is an association with both smoking and excess alcohol ingestion.

The reduced serum albumin in this patient is an indication of his poor nutritional state, partly due to poor oral intake and partly to the presence of malignancy, which may inhibit albumin synthesis. Ketonuria reflects his poor oral intake and the raised blood urea indicates dehydration.

Other causes of dysphagia include neurological conditions such as brain stem stroke, benign lesions of the oesophagus, including peptic stricture of the oesophagus, and achalasia of the cardia.

OUTCOME

The CT scan showed that the lesion was not amenable to surgical resection due to direct invasion of the mediastinum by tumour. An oesophageal tube was inserted, which allowed the patient to swallow fluid and liquidized foods. His general health deteriorated fairly rapidly and he died 2 months after initial presentation.

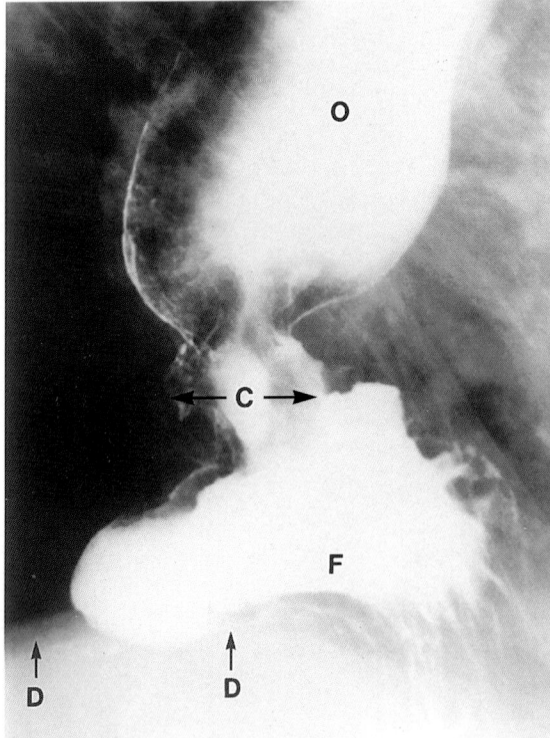

Fig. 14.3
Barium swallow showing dilated proximal oesophagus (O), oesophageal carcinoma (C), fundus of stomach (F) herniated through the diaphragm (D).

KEY POINTS

History/Examination
- Rapidly progressive dysphagia is typical of oesophageal carcinoma.

Investigations
- A combination of radiology and endoscopy is important to assess the exact nature of the lesion and to assess operability.

Outcome
- Surgical resection offers the best prospect of cure in oesophageal carcinoma, but is possible in only about 20% of cases.
- Insertion of an oesophageal tube may relieve dysphagia, providing useful palliation in terminally ill patients.

Isabella Mackenzie (75) 'Blackouts'

CASE HISTORY
Mrs Mackenzie was brought to the Accident and Emergency department by ambulance after she had 'blacked out' at home. She had been standing at the sink, helping her husband to dry the dishes, when she fell to the floor. Her husband noticed that she was pale but there were no jerking movements of her limbs and she was not incontinent. She recovered fairly rapidly, and he estimated that she had been unconscious for about 30 s.

On arrival at the hospital she was feeling much better and could not understand the 'fuss' being made over her, particularly as this had been 'just another of her turns'. Her husband confirmed that she had had several similar episodes over the last year, but she had refused to seek medical help. Mrs Mackenzie claimed that she was 'as well as one could be for 75 years'.

She lived in a detached bungalow and had four married children. She denied smoking or drinking alcohol and said that she had been taking only 'water tablets' for some 12 months.

EXAMINATION
She was alert, lucid and orientated. Her pulse rate was 40/min and regular, and blood pressure was 130/70 (supine) with no postural drop. The jugular venous pressure was normal. There were no murmurs or carotid bruits. Examination of the chest and abdomen was normal. There were no focal neurological signs.

INVESTIGATIONS
Routine investigation results

Urine	SpG 1.001	Pr neg	Glu neg	Ke neg	Blood neg
Serum	Na 140	K 3.7	HCO₃ 30	U 5.5	Cr 110
	Alb 37	Bil 5	AAT 30	AP 200	γGT 12
Blood	Hb 117	MCV 87	WCC 9.9	Plt 267	ESR 10

Additional investigations
Random blood sugar and serial cardiac enzymes were normal. The resting ECG was abnormal (Fig. 15.1), and the chest radiograph was normal.

DIAGNOSIS
Blackouts are common in the elderly. This patient's history is typical of Stokes-Adams attacks, i.e. transient episodes of loss of consciousness lasting 10–30 s with pallor and rapid return of consciousness. In this case the attacks are due to complete heart block (Fig. 15.1). Similar symptoms may occur as a result of transient tachyarrhythmias such as ventricular tachycardia, and the possibility of transient arrhythmia should be considered in any patient presenting with blackouts. If the resting ECG does not provide the diagnosis then continuous ambulatory electrocardiographic monitoring should be considered.

There are many other causes of blackouts in the elderly, the commonest being postural hypotension.

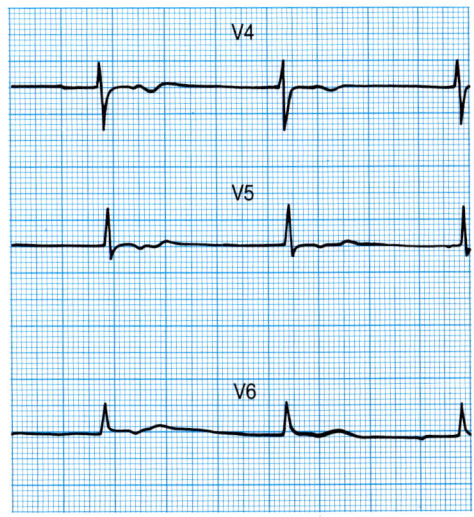

Fig. 15.1
Electrocardiograph leads V4, V5 and V6 showing complete heart block. The ventricular rate is 42/min.

OUTCOME

The patient had a permanent cardiac pacemaker inserted without further investigation (Fig. 15.2). She remained symptom-free thereafter, and her follow-up ECG shows typical pacemaker-induced electrical complexes (Fig. 15.3).

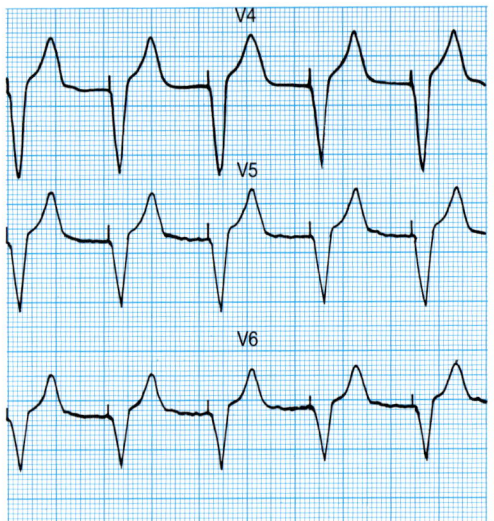

Fig. 15.3
Electrocardiograph leads V4, V5 and V6 showing pacemaker-induced complexes, i.e. regular complexes of a ventricular pattern preceded by a pacemaker 'spike'.

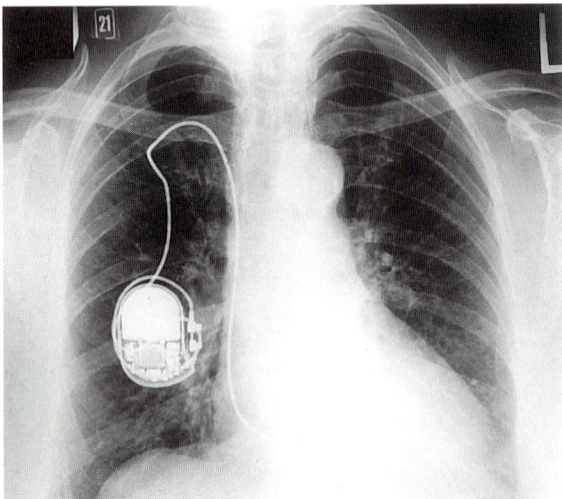

Fig. 15.2
Postero-anterior chest radiograph showing a permanent pacemaker *in situ*. The tip of the lead can be seen in the apex of the right ventricle.

KEY POINTS

History/Examination
- Transient loss of consciouness with pallor and rapid recovery is typical of a Stokes-Adams attack.
- Clinical examination of a patient with syncope should always include supine and standing blood pressure measurement to exclude postural hypotension.

Investigations
- Ambulatory electrocardiography may reveal transient arrhythmias when the resting ECG is normal.
- Complete heart block may occur without acute myocardial infarction.

Outcome
- Insertion of a pacemaker to prevent Stokes-Adams attacks is a valuable treatment irrespective of the age of the patient.

Mary Smith (71)
Tiredness, anaemia

CASE HISTORY
Mrs Smith, a widow for 7 years, had been well until a year before admission. Since that time she had become progressively lethargic and less able to look after her three-bedroomed house. An uncomplaining lady, she had recently returned to her general practitioner to see if anything could be done to help. He had found her to have a haemoglobin of 88 g/l and had requested admission for investigation. She gave no history of chest pain but had had increasing exertional dyspnoea such that going upstairs had become difficult. Her appetite was poor, and although there were no symptoms of indigestion, she had been aware for some time of an occasional niggling pain in the left side of the abdomen, spreading through to her back. There was no bowel upset or dysuria but she had been getting up on two or three occasions per night to pass water. She described an episode of 'flu' several months earlier during which she had been sweating, shivering and vomiting and for which she had been given antibiotics.

Past medical history included a pelvic floor repair 10 years previously, and a left Colles' fracture two winters ago. There was no family history of note. Both of her daughters were well and married with children; one had had tests for pregnancy diabetes. Mrs Smith was a non-smoker.

EXAMINATION
She was not undernourished but appeared pale and was dyspnoeic on minor exertion. She had slight pitting oedema at the ankles. Her pulse was 96/min and regular. There was a systolic murmur radiating into the neck, and blood pressure was 158/82. The chest was clinically normal. The abdomen was soft with no organomegaly or palpable masses. Some tenderness could be elicited in the upper abdomen to the left of the midline. Rectal examination was normal and faecal occult blood testing negative.

INVESTIGATIONS
Routine investigation results

Urine	SpG 1.010	Pr +	Glu neg	Ke neg	Blood +
Serum	Na 137	K 4.8	HCO_3 17	U 28.3	Cr 311
	Alb 32	Bil 12	AAT 23	AP 126	γGT 29
Blood	Hb 82	MCV 86	WCC 7.2	Plt 194	ESR 57

Additional investigations
A blood film showed a normochromic normocytic anaemia with burr cells (Fig. 16.1). Urine culture grew *Escherichia coli* (10^4/mm^3) and microscopy showed occasional red blood cells and pus cells. Serum calcium was 2.33 mmol/l (reference range 2.2–2.6), phosphate 1.5 mmol/l (0.7–1.2), and uric acid 0.44 mmol/l (0.18–0.42).

An ECG showed sinus rhythm of 100/min with no ischaemic features. A chest radiograph showed normal heart and lungs apart from some pulmonary venous prominence, and a plain abdominal radiograph showed opacities on both sides of the midline (Fig. 16.2).

DIAGNOSIS
This patient had chronic renal failure caused by bilateral renal obstruction as a result of staghorn calculus formation. Her tiredness, exertional dyspnoea and poor appetite were consequent upon her uraemia with the associated anaemia of impaired haemopoiesis. The blood film appearances were characteristic of

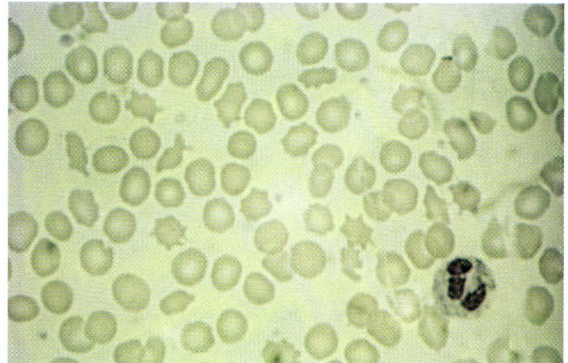

Fig. 16.1
Blood film showing numerous burr cells.

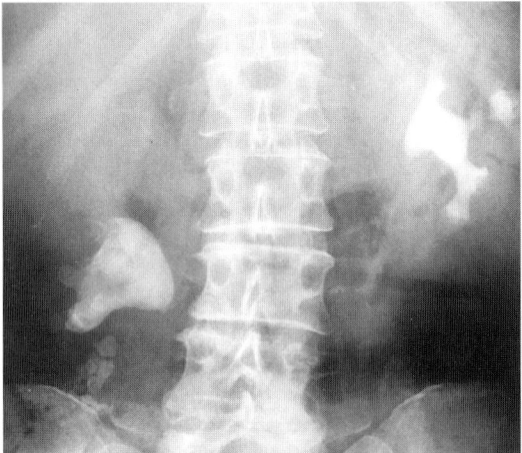

Fig. 16.2
Plain abdominal radiograph showing bilateral staghorn calculi.

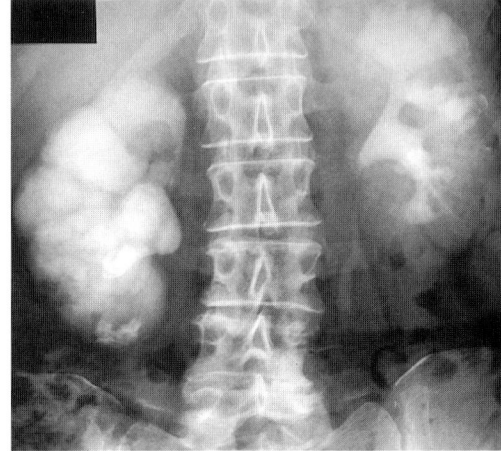

Fig. 16.3
Film from an intravenous urogram series demonstrating bilateral staghorn calculi, left hydronephrosis and persisting nephrogram indicating delayed excretion on the right.

chronic uraemia. Her 'flu'-like episode is likely to have been an episode of upper urinary tract infection in a partly obstructed renal pelvis. The current urine culture findings gave only limited contamination by *E. coli*, insufficient to signify active current infection; by convention, a microbiological diagnosis of urinary tract infection requires a growth of $>10^5$ organisms/mm^3. The absence of granular casts in the urine is evidence against there being intrinsic renal disease. Abdominal radiography was helpful in this case but only demonstrates certain types of renal calculi; in most cases of renal failure, abdominal ultrasound scanning is an extremely useful and simple technique for demonstrating renal size and the presence or absence of pelvi-ureteric dilatation.

OUTCOME

Mrs Smith had an intravenous urogram (Fig. 16.3), which demonstrated that both kidneys remained functional. She proceeded to bilateral percutaneous lithotripsy with removal of stone fragments. She was relieved of her severe anaemia and abdominal pain, and her laboratory indices showed considerable, if incomplete, improvement over the following 6 months (creatinine 172, urea 15.3, Hb 11.8). Her cardiac murmur (a simple flow murmur, often associated with severe anaemia) disappeared. Chemical analysis of the stones showed these to be of the common mixed type containing calcium, magnesium, ammonia and phosphate. A large daily fluid intake was encouraged in the long term to reduce the risk of recurrent stone formation.

KEY POINTS

History/Examination
- The clinical features of chronic renal failure are typically non-specific.
- Chronic renal failure should always be considered as a cause of a normocytic anaemia.

Investigations
- Urine examination may give important clues in the presence of renal tract pathology.
- Plain abdominal radiography may show some types of renal calculi but is usually unhelpful in chronic renal failure.
- Ultrasound scanning is an important examination for assessing renal size and demonstrating obstructive uropathy.

Outcome
- Relief of a chronic partial obstruction can sometimes result in useful improvement in renal function.

Alex Carmichael (35) Fit

CASE HISTORY
Mr Carmichael, an oil engineer, was admitted following a collapse at work. He had been preparing a report on his word processor when he suddenly blacked out and fell to the floor. A workmate reported that he had become rigid and subsequently developed generalized shaking, lasting for a few minutes. He had been incontinent of urine, and had begun to recover consciousness slowly. His workmates had called an emergency ambulance and he was brought urgently to hospital. On admission he remained drowsy. Later, when he was fully recovered and able to give a history, he described recurrent episodes of headache over the past few years. The headache was felt over the frontal region, usually developed at work and responded to simple analgesics. Recently, these headaches had been more severe. He had also noticed occasional clumsiness of his left hand while using a keyboard during the same period. His wife then mentioned that his speech had occasionally been slurred during the past few weeks.

He had had no serious previous illnesses although he had fallen from his bicycle at the age of 9 years and been knocked out; he was kept in hospital overnight for observation but no other investigations were carried out. He was married with two children, smoked 30 cigarettes per day, and drank five units of alcohol per week. There was no significant family history.

EXAMINATION
He was drowsy, but orientated in place and time. His temperature was 37.9 °C. He was obese. His pulse was 80/min and regular, and blood pressure was 140/85. Heart sounds were normal. Respiratory and abdominal examination was negative. There was no neck stiffness. He had a mild left facial weakness, but cranial nerves were otherwise normal. There was slight reduction in power in the left arm and leg for all muscle groups. Sensation was normal, tendon reflexes were present and brisk, and both plantar responses were extensor.

INVESTIGATIONS
Routine investigation results

Urine	SpG 1.020	Pr neg	Glu neg	Ke neg	Blood neg
Serum	Na 141	K 4.2	HCO₃ 26	U 4.6	Cr 90
	Alb 45	Bil 19	AAT 30	AP 103	γGT 27
Blood	Hb 161	MCV 88	WCC 11.4	Plt 259	ESR 3

Additional investigations
Blood glucose, measured by finger prick test on dry stick, was 4–6 mmol/l. A CT head scan (Fig. 17.1) was abnormal. A lumbar puncture showed that the CSF was clear and contained 2 WBC/mm³, no organisms, no growth, protein 418 mg/l (reference range < 700) and glucose 4.1 mmol/l. An electroencephalogram (EEG) (Fig. 17.2) performed 3 weeks later was normal.

DIAGNOSIS
The presenting history with loss of postural control,

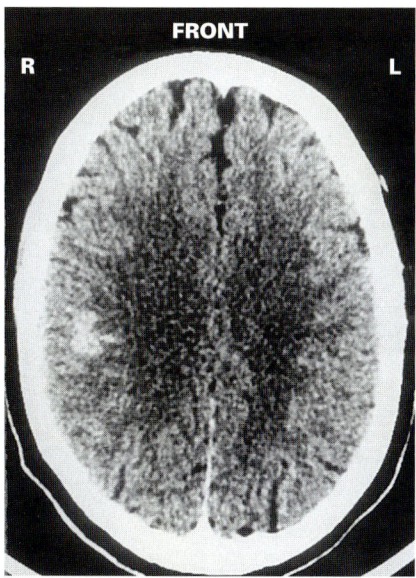

Fig. 17.1
A single transverse CT section through the head at the level of the lesion.

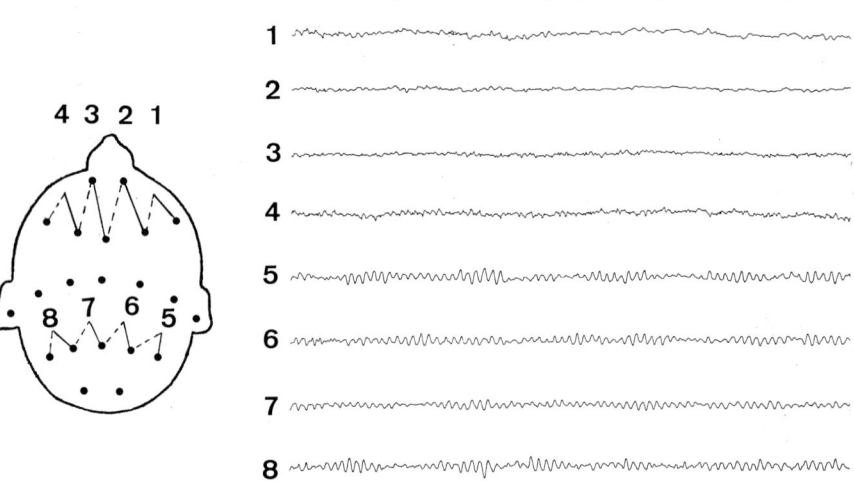

Fig. 17.2
EEG showing a normal discharge pattern.

a tonic and clonic phase, incontinence and gradual recovery of consciousness is typical of a grand mal convulsion, and the diagnosis is post-traumatic epilepsy. The finding of upgoing plantar responses during the slow recovery (post-ictal) phase is common. The preceding episodes of clumsiness may be related to focal fits.

The CT head scan shows a 1 cm calcified lesion in the right parietal cortex, which did not enhance following injection of contrast medium. This was thought to be an old calcified contusion consequent upon his previous head injury and may provide the focus for the fits. In some cases of epilepsy, fits may be precipitated by stroboscopic lighting or by watching a visual display unit.

The headaches may simply be tension headaches and unrelated to the intracranial lesion or to the epilepsy. A lumbar puncture is not routinely necessary in the investigation of epilepsy. In this case, however, as the patient was pyrexial and had an elevated white cell count, lumbar puncture was performed to exclude a small subarachnoid haemorrhage not visible on scanning, or meningitis. It would be rare for subarachnoid haemorrhage or meningitis to present with a grand mal convulsion, and the pyrexia and elevated white cell count in this case are part of the stress reaction to a convulsion.

OUTCOME

The left-sided neurological abnormalities resolved spontaneously over the following 24 h. Temporary neurological deficit after a grand mal seizure (Todd's paralysis) is not uncommon. The patient was treated with oral sodium valproate, and a CT scan 6 months later showed no changes. Mr Carmichael has continued to have occasional focal fits, with twitching of the left arm, lasting 5–15 min. He has had three further grand mal convulsions during which he lost consciousness. He remains prohibited from driving until he has completed a 2-year period free of daytime fits. He has continued his employment as an engineer, though he now limits his use of the word processor.

KEY POINTS

History/Examination
- A characteristic history is the most useful element in the diagnosis of epilepsy.
- Where episodes of collapse occur, the most useful information is often derived from a witness rather than the patient who may have no recollection of events.
- Temporary neurological deficit may be associated with the post-ictal state.

Investigations
- It is important to exclude hypoglycaemia in anyone with an acute disturbance of consciousness.
- In many cases of epilepsy, no structural lesion can be demonstrated and the EEG between attacks may also be normal.

Outcome
- Total prevention of fits may be impossible in patients with epilepsy.

Wayne Bisset (18)
Jaundice

CASE HISTORY

Mr Bisset, who worked as a gardener, became unwell over a period of 1 week complaining of tiredness, poor appetite, and nausea. His workmates were sure he must be ill as he was refusing cigarettes offered to him! Towards the end of the week, he began vomiting and called his general practitioner who noted him to be slightly jaundiced. Initially he was advised to rest in bed at home, but 2 days later he was admitted to hospital because of increasing jaundice and continuing vomiting. On enquiry, he described a darkening of his urine during the past 3 days and complained of pain and discomfort under the right ribs.

He had been previously well and was not aware of contact with jaundice. He had been in Morocco on holiday 4 months earlier. He denied taking drugs. Two years previously he had had his forearm tattooed. He normally smoked 30 cigarettes daily but had stopped since this illness began. He drank up to 10 pints of beer per week and was not taking medication.

EXAMINATION

He had a low-grade fever (37.7 °C) and was icteric (Fig. 18.1). He had a tattoo on his right forearm (Fig. 18.2). There was no pallor or lymphadenopathy and there were no stigmata of chronic liver disease. His pulse was 70/min and regular, and blood pressure was 104/60. Cardiorespiratory examination was normal. Abdominal examination revealed a slightly tender, firm liver edge palpable 2 cm below the costal margin. The remainder of the examination was normal.

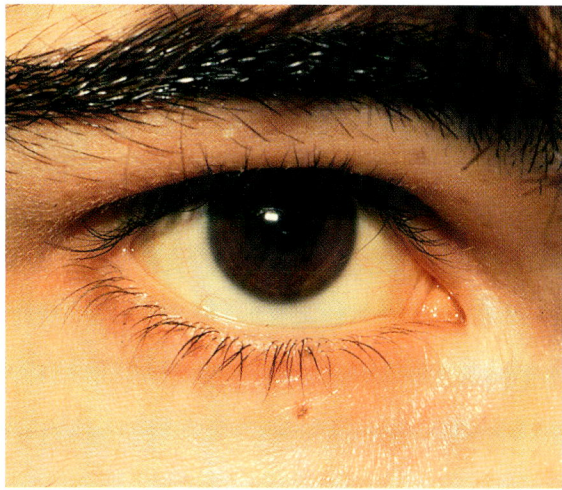

Fig. 18.1
Appearances of the eye showing icteric sclera.

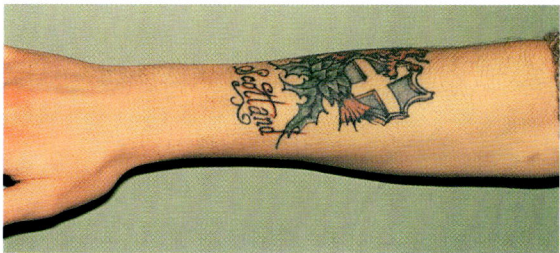

Fig. 18.2
Tattoo – a risk factor for Hepatitis B.

INVESTIGATIONS
Routine investigation results

Urine	SpG 1.003	Pr neg	Glu neg	Ke neg	Blood neg
Serum	Na 135	K 3.0	HCO$_3$ 31	U 5.0	Cr 98
	Alb 39	Bil 118	AAT 1345	AP 345	γGT 203
Blood	Hb 150	MCV 89	WCC 5.7	Plt 245	ESR 31

Additional investigations

Urinalysis showed elevated urobilinogen (+++) and bilirubin was negative. The blood film was normal and an infectious mononucleosis spot test was negative; hepatitis B surface antigen (HB$_s$Ag) was also negative. Ultrasound examination of the liver and gallbladder was normal, and stool microscopy and culture were negative. Hepatitis A IgM antibody was positive, consistent with recent or acute infection.

DIAGNOSIS

The diagnosis was acute hepatitis A infection. A

history of malaise, anorexia, nausea and vomiting followed by jaundice and dark urine is typical of viral hepatitis. Loss of taste for cigarettes is a common complaint amongst smokers with hepatitis. Hepatitis A is more likely than infectious mononucleosis, which would usually be associated with a throat infection, lymphadenopathy and skin rash. In hepatitis A, fever, icterus and tender hepatomegaly are common findings. Children and some adults may have an anicteric hepatitis, in which the serum transaminases are elevated but the bilirubin level is normal. The diagnosis is confirmed by serology. The presence of specific IgM hepatitis A antibody is diagnostic of acute or recent infection. A four-fold rise of IgG antibody would also be indicative of recent infection.

He had had a tattoo performed, which is associated with a risk of acquiring hepatitis B infection. However, the incubation period for acute hepatitis B injection is 60–180 days and it is therefore unlikely that his tattoo performed 2 years previously is relevant to his current illness. He had no other obvious risk factors for acquiring hepatitis B or C (e.g. intravenous drug misuse, blood transfusion or homosexual contact). Hepatitis due to medication was also unlikely as he had not recently taken any medication. Although the risk of acquiring hepatitis is greater in Morocco, his trip to Morocco is unlikely to be of significance as the onset of the illness is past the incubation period of hepatitis A (15–45 days) and of hepatitis E (16–60 days), both which are transmitted by the faeco-oral route.

OUTCOME

He was treated with bed rest and intravenous fluids until he stopped vomiting. Five days after admission, when the diagnosis had been confirmed and the serum transaminases showed improvement, he was discharged home. He was advised to abstain from alcohol for 1 month.

KEY POINTS

History/Examination
- Hepatitis A infection is endemic worldwide.

Investigations
- High amounts of urobilinogen in the urine and the absence of bilirubin is typical of acute hepatitis.
- Alanine and aspartate aminotransferases are typically grossly elevated reflecting hepatocellular damage.

Outcome
- Recovery from hepatitis A infection is usually complete. Unlike hepatitis B and C, there is no carrier state.

Robert Mann (47)
Collapse, diarrhoea

19

CASE HISTORY
Mr Mann, a detective constable, had felt very tired at the end of a 12 h work shift. He had been feeling nauseous all day and had had diarrhoea twice that evening. As he was leaving for home he suddenly felt light-headed and passed out. He regained consciousness a few moments later surrounded by colleagues who had already sent for an ambulance. On arrival at hospital, he immediately asked for a commode and once again had profuse diarrhoea, which, on this occasion, he noted to be very dark in colour. Systematic enquiry was unremarkable although he did admit to occasional use of proprietary antacid tablets for indigestion. There had been no vomiting.

Past medical history included rib fractures in a road accident. His father had undergone surgery for a bowel tumour. Mr Mann smoked 10 cigarettes per day and drank three to four measures of spirits twice per week. He was not taking regular medication.

EXAMINATION
He looked pale and anxious. His skin was cool and moist to the touch. His pulse was 120/min and regular, and blood pressure was 90/50. Examination of the chest was unremarkable. His abdomen was soft and non-tender with no masses or organomegaly.

Bowel sounds were particularly active. There was a characteristic smell of melaena and rectal examination was normal with a strongly positive faecal occult blood test.

INVESTIGATIONS
Routine investigation results

Urine	SpG 1.018	Pr neg	Glu neg	Ke neg	Blood neg
Serum	Na 138	K 3.9	HCO_3 23	U 16.3	Cr 68
	Alb 41	Bil 15	AAT 21	AP 87	γGT 39
Blood	Hb 127	MCV 86	WCC 11.8	Plt 388	ESR 14

Additional investigations
After resuscitation with blood transfusion he proceeded to emergency upper gastrointestinal endoscopy. A quantity of altered blood was aspirated from the stomach and an ulcer found in the first part of the duodenum with bleeding vessels at its margin (Fig. 19.1).

DIAGNOSIS
The diagnosis was bleeding duodenal ulcer resulting in collapse secondary to hypovolaemia. The ulcer is likely to have been present for some time, but appeared to have caused few symptoms. The initial haemoglobin level gave little indication of the extent of the bleeding; the elevated blood urea (with normal creatinine) occurs as a result of the breakdown of blood proteins by gut bacteria and is sometimes a useful indicator of significant gastrointestinal bleeding. It is possible that Mr Mann's recent long hours of work with consequent irregular eating habits may have contributed to the acute exacerbation of the problem.

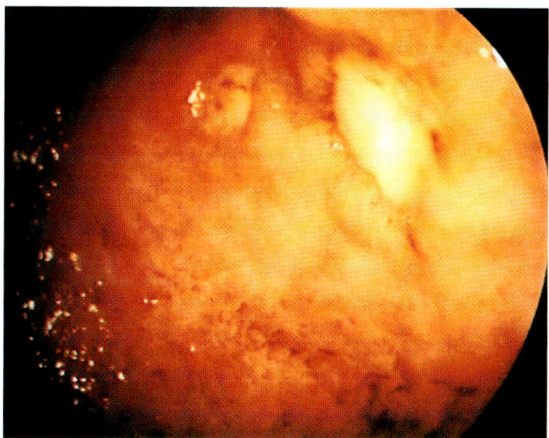

Fig. 19.1
Endoscopic view showing duodenal ulcer with peripheral bleeding points and surrounding mucosal oedema.

OUTCOME
He had a transfusion of four units of blood to correct his hypovolaemia. His pulse settled to 90/min but his haemoglobin remained low at 115 g/l. He was commenced on an intravenous H_2-receptor blocking

agent. Twelve hours after admission, he had a further large melaena and his pulse rate rose to 110/min suggesting recurrent bleeding. He had a further blood transfusion and was transferred to surgery where he underwent laparotomy with undersewing of the ulcer, vagotomy and gastroenterostomy. Recovery thereafter was uneventful.

KEY POINTS

History/Examination
- Melaena can be the major manifestation of bleeding from the upper gastrointestinal tract.
- Major blood loss can occur from a relatively asymptomatic peptic ulcer.

Investigations
- Haemoglobin level is a poor acute indicator of the extent of blood loss.
- Faecal occult blood testing is an important simple procedure.
- Upper grastrointestinal endoscopy is the most likely investigation to give a definitive diagnosis.

Outcome
- Rebleeding is not uncommon and close monitoring is essential.

Alice Ritchie (25)
Drug overdose

CASE HISTORY

Ms Ritchie, an unemployed hotel receptionist, attended the hospital Emergency Department complaining of nausea and abdominal pain. She had also had tingling in the fingers and around the mouth during the past few hours. She was in an agitated state, shouting and demanding treatment, and it took a considerable time to calm her sufficiently to obtain a history. She eventually admitted that 24 h earlier she had swallowed 24 paracetamol tablets (12 g) and two cans of strong lager after an argument with her boyfriend. She had slept for a few hours after taking the tablets, but since wakening had felt generally unwell and had eventually decided to seek medical attention. She had previously taken drug overdoses on two occasions, and had also attempted to cut her wrists in the past.

She had no other significant previous illnesses, but had been physically abused by her father in childhood. She had been taking a sleeping tablet intermittently, but did not know the name of the tablet. She denied systematic drug abuse, but had a regular alcohol intake of 30 units per week.

EXAMINATION

She was agitated and distressed, but alert and orientated. She had scars on both forearms from previous self-inflicted injuries (Fig. 20.1). During the course of examination, she developed episodes of carpopedal spasm (Fig. 20.2). There was no jaundice and no features of chronic liver disease. Her pulse was 90/min and regular, and blood pressure was 115/75. Her respiration was rapid, but breath sounds were normal with no added sounds. The heart sounds were normal. There was tenderness on deep palpation in the right upper quadrant but the liver and spleen were not palpable. Bowel sounds were normal, as was rectal examination, and the faecal occult blood test was negative. There was no focal neurological abnormality.

INVESTIGATIONS
Routine investigation results

Urine	SpG 1.020	Pr tr	Glu neg	Ke ++	Blood neg
Serum	Na 135	K 3.7	HCO_3 25	U 5	Cr 79
	Alb 48	Bil 24	AAT 120	AP 82	γGT 95
Blood	Hb 144	MCV 88	WCC 18.4	Plt 373	ESR 30

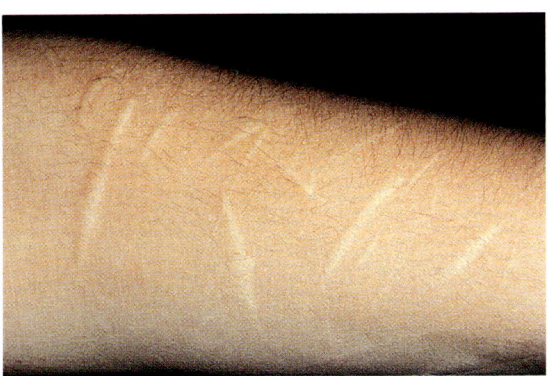

Fig. 20.1
Multiple forearm scars due to self mutilation.

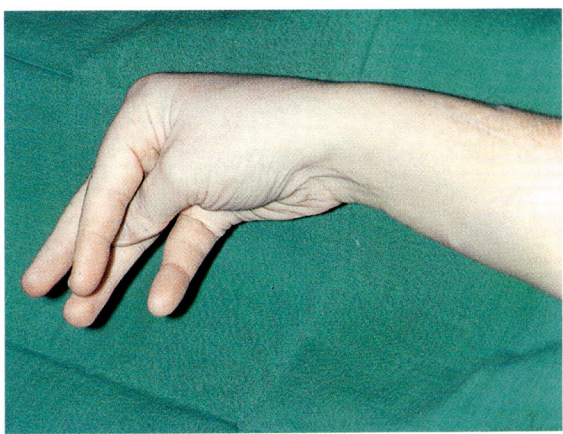

Fig. 20.2
Carpopedal spasm.

Additional investigations
Serum paracetamol level was <20 mg/l, and blood alcohol 0.3 g/l. Arterial blood gases (breathing air) were as follows:

pH	pO$_2$	pCO$_2$	sHCO$_3$
7.51	15.5	2.9	22.5

Two days after admission she became clinically jaundiced and the biochemical investigations were repeated:

Alb	Bil	AAT	AP	γGT
36	93	1173	880	113

A clotting screen at this time revealed: PT 19.8 s (reference range 12–16), APTT 38.5 s (35–45) and TCT 16.2 s (12–17).

DIAGNOSIS

This patient had developed hepatotoxicity as a consequence of paracetamol overdosage. The low levels of paracetamol measured in this patient on admission reflect late presentation. The clotting screen, particularly the prothrombin time, is a sensitive early indicator of liver damage, and in this case the liver enzymes also became markedly deranged. Hepatotoxicity results from the formation of a toxic metabolite of paracetamol generated by oxidation. This metabolite is subsequently conjugated and excreted, consuming liver glutathione stores. As these stores become overwhelmed, hepatic necrosis occurs. Toxicity can be prevented by administration of the glutathione precursors, such as N-acetyl cysteine or methionine. These are most effective if administered within 16 h of paracetamol; late presentation, as in this case, is associated with a greater risk of hepatotoxicity. In some cases, progressive liver failure may occur, with an associated high mortality.

This patient also demonstrated some of the other problems commonly seen with drug overdosage. On admission, she was distressed and agitated, and her history was difficult to obtain. In such circumstances, the history obtained may be unreliable, and further information from witnesses or friends may be important. Screening of plasma and urine for drugs may also be helpful. Tingling around the mouth and in the fingers is due to hyperventilation, which in this case resulted in carpopedal spasm (Fig. 20.2). The arterial blood gases confirm that the patient has a respiratory alkalosis which is due to hyperventilation.

OUTCOME

Gastric lavage was performed as there was concern that she may have ingested drugs more recently than she admitted. An infusion of N-acetyl cysteine was also given; although it was more than 16 h since ingestion, recent evidence suggests that there may be benefit in treating even at this stage.

In this case, although abnormalities of liver function developed, progressive liver failure did not occur. Ms Ritchie was kept under observation for a further week, during which her liver function gradually returned to normal. She agreed to psychiatric treatment and was also assessed for social support.

KEY POINTS

History/Examination
- In cases of self-poisoning, the history may be unreliable.

Investigations
- Serious liver damage due to paracetamol is often delayed to 48–72 h after ingestion.
- Serum levels of the ingested drug must be interpreted in relation to time of ingestion.

Outcome
- Monitoring of the patient until significant liver damage can be excluded is desirable.
- Psychiatric assessment of patients with deliberate self-poisoning is important.

Alison Stewart (22)
21 Dysuria/loin pain

CASE HISTORY
Miss Stewart, a student nurse, was admitted to hospital with a 3-day history of fever, sweating, headaches and severe aching pain in the right loin. During this time she had noticed discomfort on passing urine and had been passing urine more frequently than normal.

In the past, she had had three urinary tract infections requiring antibiotics but she had not previously been admitted to hospital with these episodes. Her general health had otherwise been good. She was single and had a steady boyfriend. She was a non-smoker and took alcohol only on occasions.

EXAMINATION
On admission she was flushed, febrile (38.5°C) and distressed with pain. Her pulse was 110/min and regular, and blood pressure was 120/70. Apart from moderate tenderness over the right renal angle, the remainder of the examination was normal.

INVESTIGATIONS
Routine investigation results

Urine	SpG 1.05	Pr +++	Glu neg	Ke +	Blood ++
Serum	Na 134	K 3.9	HCO$_3$ 23	U 6.0	Cr 59
	Alb 36	Bil 9	AAT 11	AP 89	γGT 10
Blood	Hb 129	MCV 79	WCC 18.9	Plt 330	ESR 65

Additional investigations
A blood film revealed a neutrophil leucocytosis. A mid-stream sample of urine (MSSU) contained pus cells (+++) and rod-shaped organisms (>10^5/mm^3). A Gram stain confirmed that these were Gram-negative bacilli (Fig. 21.1), and culture showed them to be *Escherichia coli*. Blood cultures were sterile.

A plain abdominal radiograph was normal. Renal ultrasound indicated that the right kidney was large,

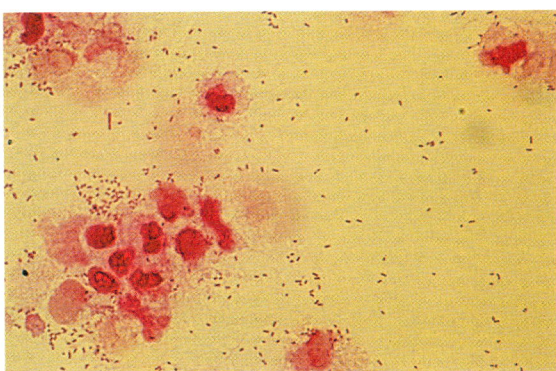

Fig. 21.1
Gram stain of spun urine specimen showing pus cells and Gram-negative bacilli.

and an intravenous urogram (IVU) revealed a right-sided duplex kidney and ureter (Fig. 21.2). There was no evidence of urinary tract obstruction.

DIAGNOSIS
Dysuria and frequency commonly occur as a result of cystitis in young women. The presence of fever and loin pain in this case suggested the diagnosis of pyelonephritis. Urinary tract infection is a common cause of bacteraemia in young adult women, and may occur with few urinary symptoms. Recurrent urinary tract infections are usually due to reinfection by the periurethral flora, or less commonly to relapsing or persistent infection of the upper urinary tract, often as a result of an underlying structural abnormality, such as duplex kidneys or ureters.

Renal ultrasound is a valuable, non-invasive method to demonstrate renal size and obstruction to the collecting system. Intravenous urography provides some information on renal function and is useful to visualize ureteric anatomy, in this case revealing a duplex right kidney.

OUTCOME
Miss Stewart was given appropriate analgesia and, once the MSSU and blood cultures samples had been

obtained, an intravenous antibiotic was commenced. In view of the structural abnormality of the urinary tract and the resulting high likelihood of further infections, she was advised to take long-term antibiotic therapy.

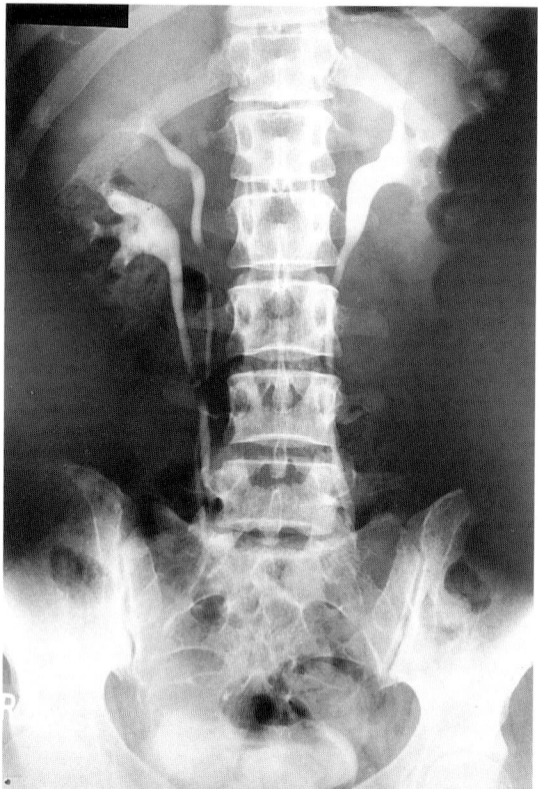

Fig. 21.2
A 20 min radiograph from an IVU series showing a right duplex system.

KEY POINTS

History/Examination
- A history of recurrent urinary tract infection is an indication for investigation of structural abnormalities of the urinary tract.

Investigations
- The presence of pus cells and organisms in a fresh sample of urine is diagnostic of urinary infection.
- Renal ultrasound and intravenous urography are complementary investigations in the assessment of the urinary tract.

Outcome
- Anatomical abnormalities of the urinary tract predispose to recurrent infections.

Grace Mortimer (59)
Jaundice, weight loss

CASE HISTORY
Mrs Mortimer, a care assistant in a residential home for the elderly, had been finding her work more tiring over the previous month, and was considering retirement. When her general practitioner attended the home to see an elderly patient, he immediately noted that Mrs Mortimer looked unwell with perhaps a yellowish tinge to her sclerae. He asked her to call at the surgery the following day for blood tests and on receiving the results arranged for her direct admission to the on-call medical ward. On admission, further enquiry revealed a recent loss of appetite, slight epigastric discomfort, normal bowel habit and darkening of her urine. She admitted to weight loss of about 5 kg in the previous 2 months.

Past medical history included hysterectomy for menorrhagia at age 44 years, right mastectomy and radiotherapy for breast carcinoma at age 49 years, and left-sided sciatica 3 years ago. Her father had died of ischaemic heart disease aged 75 years; her mother was well, in her mid-eighties. Mrs Mortimer had two married daughters who were both well. She had smoked 10 cigarettes per day until her current illness and drank little alcohol. Her only medication was tamoxifen (20 mg/day).

EXAMINATION
She was lean and pale with icteric sclerae (Fig. 22.1),

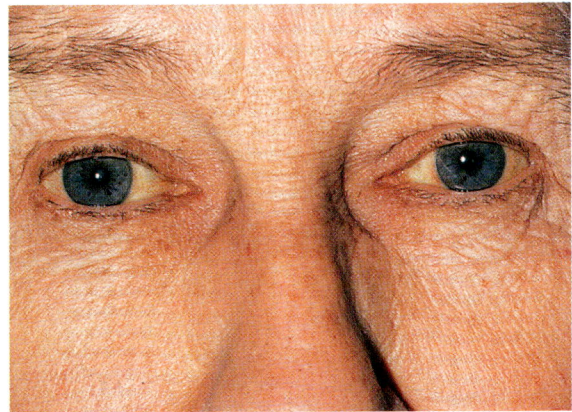

Fig. 22.1
Icteric sclerae.

and was apyrexial. There was a trace of ankle oedema. Her pulse was 80/min, and blood pressure was 134/76. The right mastectomy scar was noted. The trachea was deviated to the right and bronchial breath sounds and coarse crackles were audible over the upper part of the right lung. The heart sounds were normal. There was a fullness of the right upper quadrant on inspection and abdominal palpation revealed a firm irregular mass extending 7 cm below the right costal margin. This was slightly tender but there was no associated bruit. There were no other abdominal abnormalities.

INVESTIGATIONS
Routine investigation results

Urine	SpG 1.015	Pr tr	Glu neg	Ke neg	Blood neg
Serum	Na 135	K 3.5	HCO3 22	U 4.1	Cr 87
	Alb 31	Bil 64	AAT 144	AP 291	γGT 393
Blood	Hb 104	MCV 89	WCC 5.4	Plt 198	ESR 37

Additional investigations
Urine was positive for bilirubin. The prothrombin time was 17.2 s against a control value of 14.3 s. A chest radiograph showed the previous mastectomy and opacification of the upper right lung field (Fig. 22.2). An abdominal ultrasound scan revealed hepatomegaly with multiple echo-dense lesions suggestive of metastases (Fig. 22.3). There was no evidence of dilatation of the extrahepatic biliary system. Fine-needle liver aspiration under ultrasound control yielded malignant cells with appearances very similar to those in the breast carcinoma removed 10 years earlier.

DIAGNOSIS
This patient was suffering from a series of non-specific systemic complaints, namely lethargy, anorexia, weight loss and anaemia. The abdominal pain, hepatomegaly and development of jaundice indicated hepatic involvement in the underlying disease process.

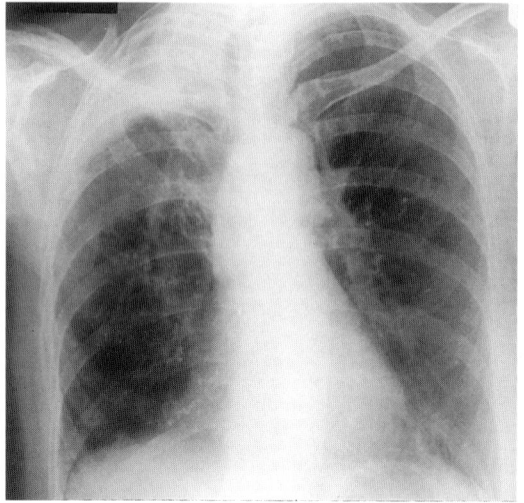

Fig. 22.2
Chest radiograph showing right mastectomy and an area of post-irradiation fibrosis in the right upper zone. Note the tracheal deviation.

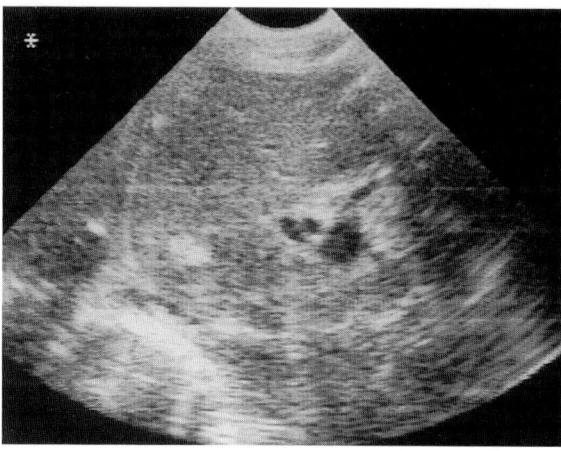

Fig. 22.3
Ultrasound scan section through the liver showing multiple echo-dense areas typical of metastatic carcinoma.

Ultrasound scanning quickly revealed the nature of the problem to be metastatic carcinoma, as had been suggested on abdominal examination. Cytological examination of a liver aspirate confirmed the likelihood that the primary lesion was her earlier breast cancer, a condition that is notorious for late recurrence.

The biochemical findings had indicated elements of hepatocellular disease (elevated AAT and low albumin) and of biliary obstruction (elevated bilirubin, alkaline phosphatase and γ-glutamyl transpeptidase). The hepatocellular element signifies metastatic liver infiltration and the obstruction, intrahepatic cholestasis; evidence of extrahepatic biliary obstruction, when present, is usually apparent on ultrasound scanning. The chest findings were due to radiation fibrosis following her radiotherapy; this had also produced the tracheal deviation and the opacity at the right apex on the chest radiograph.

OUTCOME

The patient's condition rapidly deteriorated with progressive weight loss, anorexia, vomiting and upper abdominal discomfort. Latterly her jaundice deepened, her conscious level deteriorated and she died from the combined effects of carcinomatosis and hepatic failure only 2 months after her jaundice was first detected.

KEY POINTS

History/Examination
- Neoplastic disease often presents with non-specific symptoms and weight loss.
- Breast carcinoma can recur many years after treatment of the primary disease.

Investigations
- The pattern of abnormality in liver function tests is of great diagnostic value.
- Ultrasound scanning can usually rapidly differentiate between intrahepatic and extrahepatic biliary obstruction.

23 Joanne Fairley (21)
Wheeze, breathlessness

CASE HISTORY
Miss Fairley, a hairdresser, was admitted as an emergency at 9.30 am. She had wakened 4 h earlier with a coughing episode, rapidly followed by wheezing and a feeling that she 'couldn't breathe'. She had a history of recurrent attacks of wheezing since age 10 years. She normally used inhaled corticosteroids regularly and a bronchodilator inhaler when wheezy, but her inhalers had run out some days previously.

She had suffered from eczema since childhood, and had one sister who was asthmatic. She lived with her parents and sister and kept a golden retriever. She smoked 10 cigarettes daily.

EXAMINATION
She was distressed and tachypnoeic (respiratory rate 35 breaths/min) and was using accessory muscles of respiration. Her fingers and tongue were cyanosed, and she was commenced immediately on oxygen therapy before being examined (Fig. 23.1). Her pulse rate was 130/min, and blood pressure was 130/80 during expiration and 100/80 during inspiration. Her chest was hyperinflated and resonant on percussion, and she had bilateral expiratory wheezes. Abdominal examination was difficult because breathlessness made it impossible to lie flat. Neurological examination was normal. Her peak expiratory flow rate was less than 60 l/min.

INVESTIGATIONS
Routine investigation results

Urine	SpG 1020	Pr neg	Glu neg	Ke tr	Blood neg
Serum	Na 141	K 5.0	HCO_3 23	U 5.5	Cr 89
	Alb 39	Bil 13	AAT 12	AP 99	γGT 30
Blood	Hb 155	MCV 87	WCC 24.6	Plt 505	ESR 35

Additional investigations
Arterial blood gases measured while she was breathing 60% oxygen were as follows:

pH	pO_2	pCO_2	$sHCO_3$
7.49	20.5	3.4	26

The chest radiograph is shown in Fig. 23.2. Total serum IgE was 833 IU/ml (reference range 0–100), and there were raised levels of IgE specific to cat epithelium, dog dander, egg white, grass pollen and house dust mite.

DIAGNOSIS
The previous history of recurrent wheezing and family history of asthma are important, and together with the acute history and physical signs suggest a diagnosis of acute severe asthma. The acute attack may have been precipitated by omission of treatment or exposure to allergen, though in many cases no obvious precipitating event can be identified.

Clinical signs indicating the severity of the attack include cyanosis, tachycardia and the pulse pressure reduction during inspiration (pulsus paradoxus). In

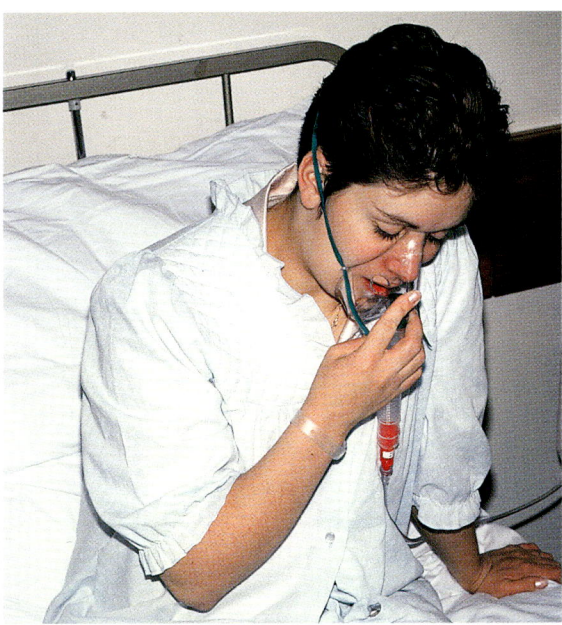

Fig. 23.1
Appearances of the patient during acute severe asthma. Note the upright posture, allowing use of accessory muscles of respiration.

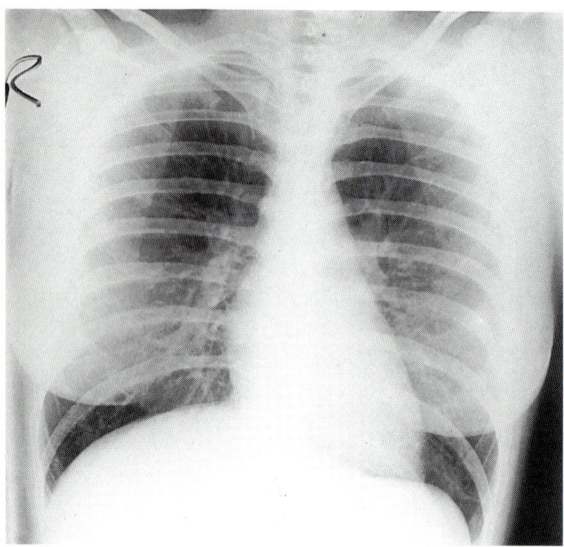

Fig. 23.2
Chest radiograph showing hyperinflation of the lungs. There is no evidence of pneumothorax.

extremely severe asthma, patients may be unable to speak, and wheeze and even breath sounds may become completely inaudible as air entry to the chest decreases. Blood gases were measured to assess the adequacy of ventilation as indicated by the pCO_2. In this case, the mild reduction in pCO_2 suggests that alveolar ventilation is adequate, though if the attack were to continue untreated, carbon dioxide retention may eventually supervene, leading to worsening hypoxia and eventually to death. The chest radiograph was performed to exclude the presence of pneumothorax, a potentially fatal complication of acute severe asthma.

OUTCOME

She was treated with 60% oxygen, inhaled nebulized bronchodilators, and intravenous and oral corticosteroids. Her clinical condition and peak flow rate, which were monitored regularly, gradually improved over the following 72 h (Fig. 23.3), and she was discharged from hospital after 5 days. She completed a 10-day course of oral corticosteroids and thereafter continued on a regular inhaled corticosteroid and used a bronchodilator inhaler when required. She was advised to stop smoking and to avoid contact with the dog.

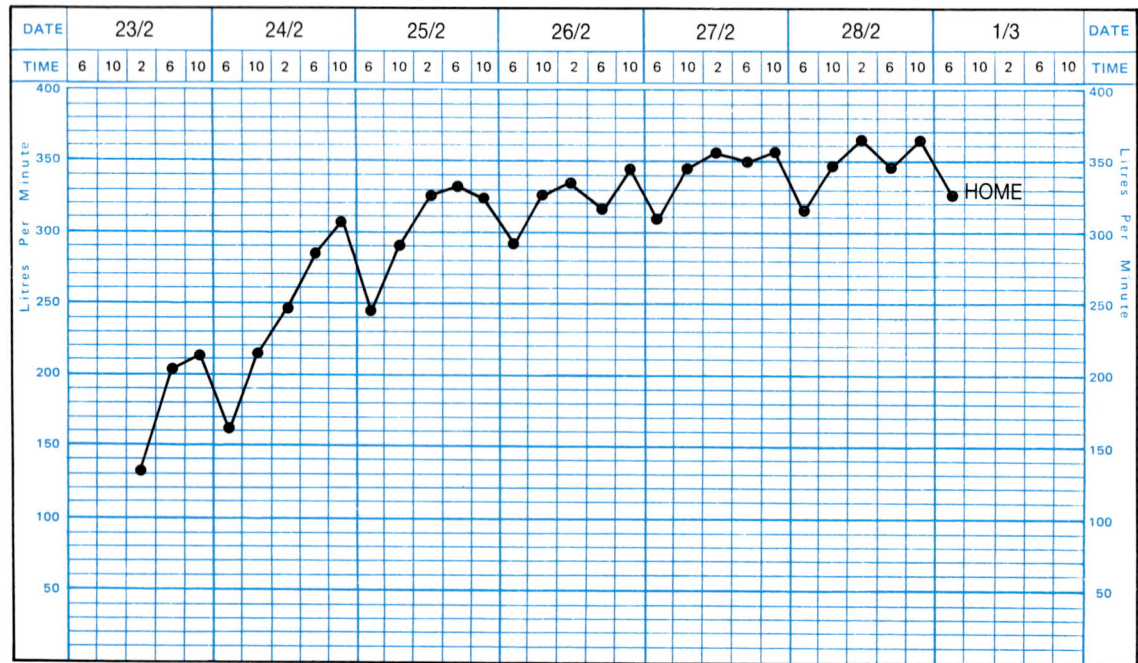

Fig. 23.3
Peak expiratory flow chart showing improvement over the first 72 h of admission.

KEY POINTS

History/Examination
- Acute severe asthma may occur without any obvious precipitating cause.
- Measurement of the peak expiratory flow rate is important in assessing the severity of asthma.

Investigations
- A chest radiograph and blood gas estimation are important early investigations.
- Measurement of blood gases should not await the institution of treatment with oxygen.

Outcome
- If there is evidence of hypercapnia, indicating ventilatory failure, then assisted ventilation should be urgently considered.
- Prophylactic treatment is important to prevent recurrent attacks of asthma.

James Lewis (24)
Bloody diarrhoea

CASE HISTORY
Mr Lewis was admitted to hospital with a 3-week history of progressively worsening frequent watery diarrhoea. He described passing fresh blood and mucus mixed with loose stool. The diarrhoea had been associated with right-sided abdominal pain which he described as 'coming and going'. He had been feeling generally unwell with some loss of appetite and had lost 8 kg in weight over the past 3 months.

He had experienced one similar transient episode of bloody diarrhoea about 3 years earlier. This had lasted for a week and had settled without treatment. Apart from recurrent mouth ulcers, for which he was treated with local analgesics, he had no other past medical history of note. His mother, who was a nurse, also had 'bowel problems', although he was unclear as to their cause. He smoked 10 cigarettes daily but did not drink any alcohol.

EXAMINATION
He was flushed and pyrexial (37.7 °C). He had several painful oral aphthous ulcers (Fig. 24.1) but no skin rashes, finger clubbing, pallor or lymphadenopathy. His pulse was 100/min and regular, and blood pressure was 104/74. The jugular venous pulse was not visible. Cardiac and respiratory examination was normal. Abdominal examination revealed some tenderness in both iliac fossae but no guarding. Bowel sounds were active, and rectal examination showed moderate amounts of fresh blood and mucus. The remainder of the examination was normal.

INVESTIGATIONS
Routine investigation results

Urine	SpG 1.003	Pr neg	Glu neg	Ke neg	Blood neg
Serum	Na 130	K 3.4	HCO$_3$ 31	U 4.9	Cr 78
	Alb 29	Bil 20	AAT 19	AP 67	γGT 21
Blood	Hb 100	MCV 68	WCC 10.9	Plt 356	ESR 89

Additional investigations
The blood film revealed a hypochromic microcytic anaemia. Blood cultures were sterile, and stool microscopy and culture showed no pathogens. Sigmoidoscopy to 15 cm showed an inflamed rectal mucosa with contact bleeding (Fig. 24.2). Rectal biopsy histology revealed changes consistent with an

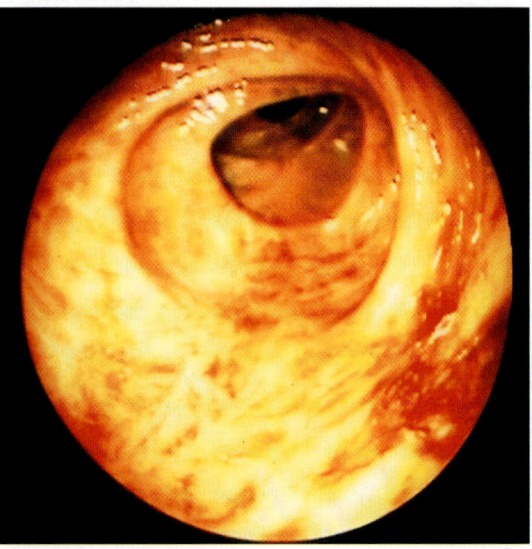

Fig. 24.2
Sigmoidoscopic appearance showing oedematous mucosa with contact bleeding.

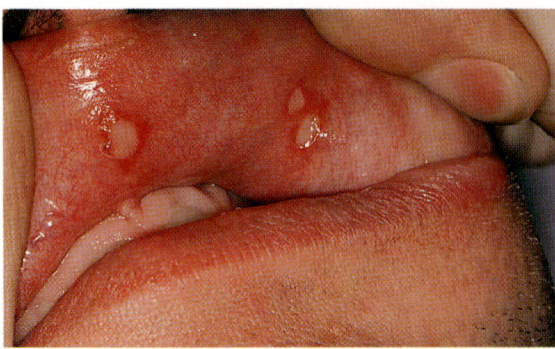

Fig. 24.1
Oral aphthous ulceration.

acute exacerbation of ulcerative colitis. Double-contrast barium enema (Fig. 24.3) was abnormal.

DIAGNOSIS

The history of profuse and prolonged diarrhoea with or without blood, constitutional symptoms such as weight loss and a possible family history of bowel disease suggest the diagnosis of inflammatory bowel disease in this patient. Recurrent aphthous ulceration is also a common feature of inflammatory bowel disease. The possibility of an infective diarrhoea (most commonly salmonellosis or shigellosis) must be considered and the negative stool microscopy and culture excluded this. Proctitis, i.e. colonic inflammation confined to the rectum, usually leads to recurrent episodes of bloody diarrhoea but is not associated with systemic symptoms and chronic morbidity.

In this patient, the barium enema confirmed that the entire colon was abnormal, but the distal ileum was normal, supporting the diagnosis of ulcerative colitis. The low haemoglobin and low albumin are important indicators of chronic inflammation, while the fast ESR reflects the current disease activity.

OUTCOME

He was treated initially with intravenous fluids, hydrocortisone foam suppositories and oral prednisolone, and improved gradually over the following 2 weeks. He was discharged home on a maintenance dose of mesalazine (a 5-aminosalicylate) and decremental doses of oral prednisolone.

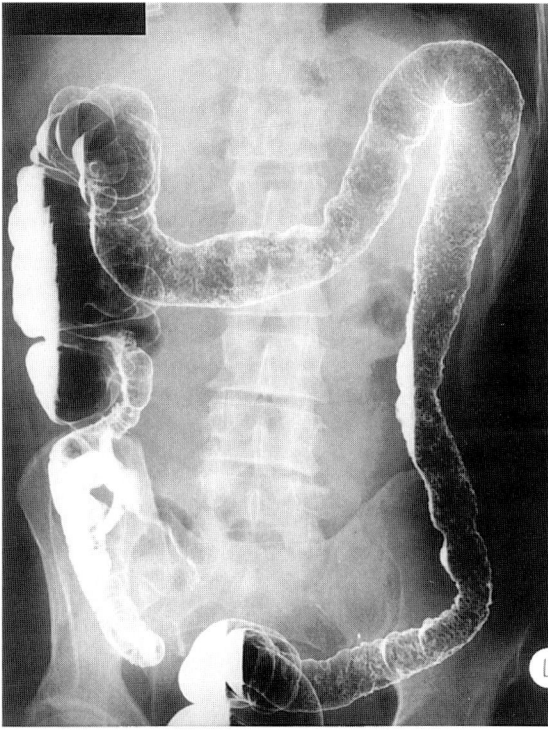

Fig. 24.3
Double-contrast barium enema showing extensive superficial mucosal ulceration throughout the colon. The distal ileum is normal.

KEY POINTS

History/Examination
- Diarrhoea may be due to infection or may be the presenting feature of inflammatory bowel disease.

Investigations
- Stool microscopy and culture are important to exclude infection.
- Sigmoidoscopy or colonoscopy with biopsy are required to establish the diagnosis of inflammatory bowel disease.
- Double-contrast barium enema is used to estimate the extent of disease.

Outcome
- The extent of disease dictates the need for local or systemic maintenance treatment.

Mary McBride (53)
Abdominal pain, weight loss

CASE HISTORY

Mrs McBride had always had a considerable weight problem despite many different reducing diets and intermittent attendance at slimming clubs over 20 years. During the year before presentation, she was surprised that at last she was managing to lose weight without much difficulty. For 2 months she had been aware of intermittent discomfort in the epigastric region, which gradually became more persistent and severe, radiating through to her back and disturbing sleep. The pain was worse after eating. By the time she consulted her general practitioner she had lost almost 30 kg in weight, was in constant pain and had no appetite or energy. She had not vomited but had been having loose stools.

She had no previous history of abdominal symptoms but had suffered from backache and arthritic knees, for which she took a non-steroidal anti-inflammatory drug. She had had hypothyroidism diagnosed 11 years earlier, and was on thyroxine replacement therapy. Co-dydramol, and more recently pethidine, had been of limited help in relieving her abdominal pain. There was a family history of obesity. She smoked 15 cigarettes per day but did not drink any alcohol.

EXAMINATION

She was overweight at 77 kg but she had loose skin indicating weight loss. She had no pallor, jaundice or lymphadenopathy. Her pulse was 72/min and regular, and blood pressure was 144/92. The heart sounds were normal and examination of the chest was unremarkable. There was tenderness on epigastric palpation but abdominal exmination was otherwise normal. Rectal examination was normal and faecal occult blood testing was negative. There were no neurological abnormalities.

INVESTIGATIONS
Routine investigation results

Urine	SpG 1.008	Pr tr	Glu neg	Ke neg	Blood neg
Serum	Na 142	K 3.5	HCO$_3$ 25	U 3.6	Cr 72
	Alb 32	Bil 22	AAT 14	AP 132	γGT 18
Blood	Hb 139	MCV 82	WCC 10.6	Plt 255	ESR 21

Additional investigations

Serum calcium was 1.94 mmol/l (reference range 2.20–2.60), serum amylase 188 U/l (< 340), random blood glucose 7.0 mmol/l (< 8.0), serum thyroxine 162 nmol/l (70–150) and TSH 0.41 mUl/l (0.35–3.30).

Chest and plain abdominal radiographs were normal. An abdominal ultrasound scan showed a number of calculi in the gallbladder and normal calibre of the biliary tree. The pancreatic head was prominent but within the normal range, and the liver, kidneys and spleen were normal. Barium meal was normal. An abdominal CT scan showed irregularity of the head of pancreas extending posteriorly into the uncinate process (Fig. 25.1). The tail of pancreas was atrophic and there was no retroperitoneal lymphadenopathy. Endoscopic retrograde cholangiopancreatography (ERCP) confirmed that the bile ducts were normal. There was no filling of the pancreatic duct despite apparently good position of the cannula.

DIAGNOSIS

At this stage in the investigations, the diagnosis remained uncertain although there was a suspicious lesion in the head of pancreas. Fine-needle aspiration under ultrasound control was unsuccessful in obtaining diagnostically useful cells. In view of her progressive symptoms, Mrs McBride proceeded to laparotomy, at which a firm mass was found in the head of pancreas adherent to the adjacent aorta; frozen-section histology confirmed malignancy and formal histology subsequently showed typical features

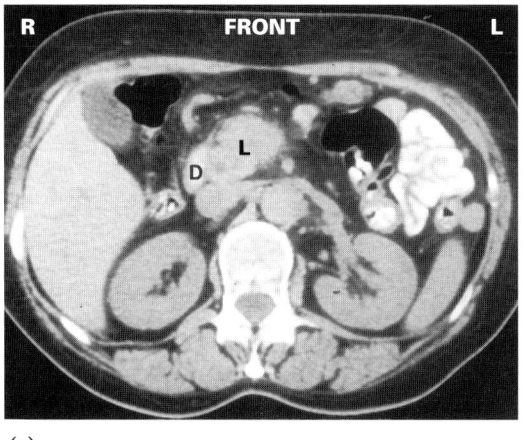 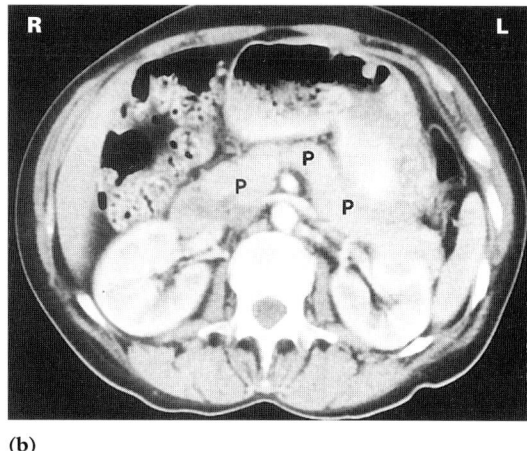

Fig. 25.1
(a) Single transverse CT section through the abdomen at the level of L1 showing lesion in the head of pancreas (L), and radiographic contrast in the second part of the duodenum (D). Note atrophy of the tail of pancreas. (b) Similar CT scan section (contrast enhanced) from another patient for comparison showing a normal pancreas (P).

of poorly differentiated adenocarcinoma. The loose stools were a reflection of exocrine pancreatic insufficiency. The low serum calcium, even when corrected for the subnormal albumin concentration (by adding 0.025 mmol/l for every gram of albumin below 40 g/l), and elevated alkaline phosphatase suggest a degree of osteomalacia consequent upon malabsorption of calcium and vitamin D. The low albumin may be related to malabsorption, or to reduced hepatic albumin synthesis as a systemic manifestation of malignant disease. While there was no obstruction to biliary drainage in this patient, jaundice is often an associated feature in disease of the head of pancreas. The thyroid function tests were satisfactory for someone on thyroxine replacement therapy, and overtreatment was not contributing to the weight loss.

OUTCOME

The lesion was unresectable at laparotomy in view of its local spread. Mrs McBride was given pancreatic enzyme supplements and proceeded to combined chemotherapy and radiotherapy, which was complicated by the development of radiation-induced pancreatitis. She initially had some relief from her symptoms and regained a little weight but 4 months after presentation her condition deteriorated again and she died of a supervening bronchopneumonia.

KEY POINTS

History/Examination
- Major unexplained weight loss usually indicates serious underlying disease.
- Epigastric or back pain, weight loss and loose stools suggest pancreatic disease.

Investigations
- The pancreas is a difficult organ to image.
- Despite the use of all available imaging techniques, laparotomy is sometimes a necessary investigative procedure.

Outcome
- Pancreatic carcinoma is often unresectable at diagnosis and has a poor prognosis.

Jane Pilcher (85)
Breathlessness, pallor

CASE HISTORY

Mrs Pilcher, a widow, called her general practitioner complaining of breathlessness, which she had first noticed on walking to her local shop about 6 weeks previously. For 2 weeks prior to seeking assistance, she had also had ankle swelling occurring as the day progressed. However, for 2 or 3 months before this she had been feeling tired and listless. She had been sleeping and eating poorly, and complained of a sore tongue, but denied other symptoms. Her daughter had commented that she looked tired and pale.

She had never had any major illnesses, and had worked as a waitress until aged 65 years. She was a non-smoker, did not drink alcohol, and lived alone, next door to her daughter.

EXAMINATION

She was pale, mildly jaundiced and had a smooth tongue (Fig. 26.1). She had bruising of both upper and lower limbs. Her pulse was 110/min and the jugular venous pulse was elevated to 5 cm above the sternal angle. Her blood pressure was 140/95. The heart sounds were normal and there was an ejection systolic murmur audible in the aortic area with radiation to the neck. She had mild bilateral ankle oedema. The respiratory system and abdominal examinations were normal. Rectal examination was normal and the faecal occult blood test was negative. There were no focal neurological abnormalities, other than absent ankle jerks.

INVESTIGATIONS
Routine investigation results

Urine	SpG 1.010	Pr neg	Glu neg	Ke neg	Blood neg
Serum	Na 145	K 3.9	HCO_3 23	U 9.0	Cr 123
	Alb 35	Bil 32	AAT 51	AP 53	γGT 12
Blood	Hb 60	MCV 115	WCC 3.5	Plt 19	ESR 35

Additional investigations

The blood film (Fig. 26.2) was abnormal. Serum B_{12} was 94 ng/l (reference range 170–1000), serum folate 2.7 μg/l (2.5–14.0) and red cell folate 160 μg/l (150–650). Thyroid function tests were normal. Intrinsic factor antibody and parietal cell antibody tests were both positive.

DIAGNOSIS

The diagnosis is marrow failure consequent upon severe pernicious anaemia. The symptoms of anaemia,

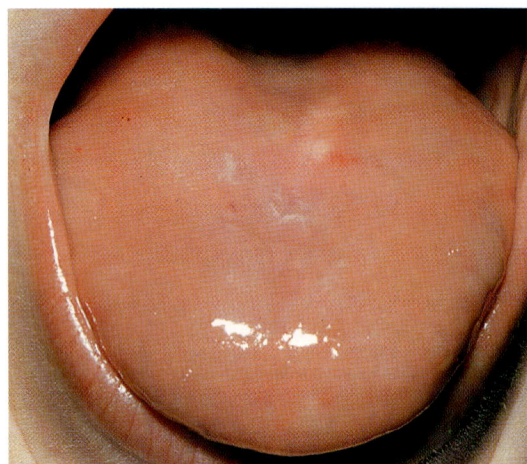

Fig. 26.1
Smooth tongue.

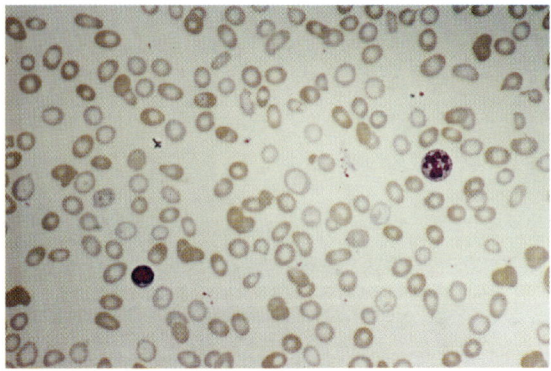

Fig. 26.2
Haematoxylin and eosin stained blood film showing oval macrocytes, a hypersegmented neutrophil and paucity of platelets.

tiredness and general malaise are vague and insidious. The ankle swelling and elevation of the jugular venous pulse suggests that Mrs Pilcher has developed cardiac failure. The mild jaundice is due to haemolysis of red cells and bruising is related to her thrombocytopenia. All elements in the peripheral blood film are depressed, and the high MCV and presence of oval macrocytes and hypersegmented neutrophils in the blood film is typical of vitamin B_{12} or folic acid deficiency. The serum B_{12} level is low and the presence of intrinsic factor antibody suggests that this is likely to be due to Addisonian pernicious anaemia, in which the gastric mucosa is atrophic and there is hypochlorhydria and deficiency of intrinsic factor secretion by the gastric parietal cells. The diagnosis can be confirmed by the Schilling test, in which the absorption of vitamin B_{12} is measured with and without the administration of intrinsic factor. This allows pernicious anaemia to be distinguished from vitamin B_{12} malabsorption due to other causes, such as disease of the terminal ileum and blind loop syndrome in which addition of intrinsic factor does not improve absorption.

Absent ankle jerks are common in the elderly and are often of no significance. Mrs Pilcher had no other clinical signs to suggest subacute combined degeneration of the cord, which occurs in some patients with vitamin B_{12} deficiency. Clinical features suggesting this diagnosis would be loss of position and vibration sense together with weakness and, in the late stages, spasticity. These neurological abnormalities may precede the haematological features of vitamin B_{12} deficiency. Thyroid function tests were checked as other organ-specific autoimmune diseases are often associated with pernicious anaemia.

OUTCOME

She was treated with daily injections of hydroxocobalamin for 5 days together with oral potassium supplements. She required a small dose of loop diuretic in view of cardiac failure consequent upon the anaemia. By 6 weeks post-treatment, her haemoglobin, platelet count and white cell count had returned to normal. The symptoms and signs of cardiac failure had resolved, the murmur disappeared, and the diuretic was discontinued. Monthly injections of hydroxocobalamin were commenced and will be continued lifelong.

KEY POINTS

History/Examination
- Consider anaemia as a cause of malaise and cardiac failure in the elderly.

Investigations
- Vitamin B_{12} or folate deficiency can be suspected from the blood film.

Outcome
- Blood tranfusion in patients with severe pernicious anaemia should be avoided where possible as it may precipitate severe cardiac failure.
- Lifelong replacement therapy with hydroxocobalamin is necessary in pernicious anaemia.

Ali Afzal (16)
Chest pain

CASE HISTORY

Mr Afzal became acutely unwell with fever, malaise and muscle pains. Thinking he had 'flu, he missed school and remained in bed. However, the following day he felt more unwell with a dull headache and developed sharp anterior chest pain. The pain was severe but seemed to be partially relieved when he sat up in bed and leaned forward. His mother became concerned and called his general practitioner, who noted a faint macular rash over his trunk, arms and legs, and decided to admit him to hospital for further investigation.

He had previously been well, and had been playing rugby 2 days before his illness. He denied smoking and took no alcohol or medication. There was no family history of diabetes, hypertension or heart disease.

EXAMINATION

He was distressed with chest pain and was febrile (37.7°C). There was a faint macular rash over his trunk and legs. His pulse was 100/min and regular, and blood pressure was 110/80. His jugular venous pulse was not raised and there was no peripheral oedema. He had normal heart sounds and a pericardial rub which varied in intensity with varying posture. Respiratory and abdominal examinations were normal. There was no neck stiffness and no focal neurological abnormality.

INVESTIGATIONS
Routine investigation results

Urine	SpG 1.005	Pr neg	Glu neg	Ke neg	Blood neg
Serum	Na 134	K 4.2	HCO$_3$ 24	U 3.6	Cr 67
	Alb 37	Bil 9	AAT 11	AP 130	γGT 28
Blood	Hb 147	MCV 86	WCC 3.4	Plt 342	ESR 45

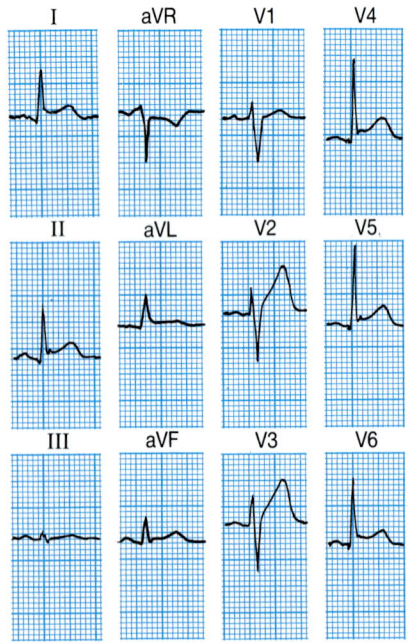

Fig. 27.1
ECG showng ST elevation, concave upwards, in all leads except aVR and V1.

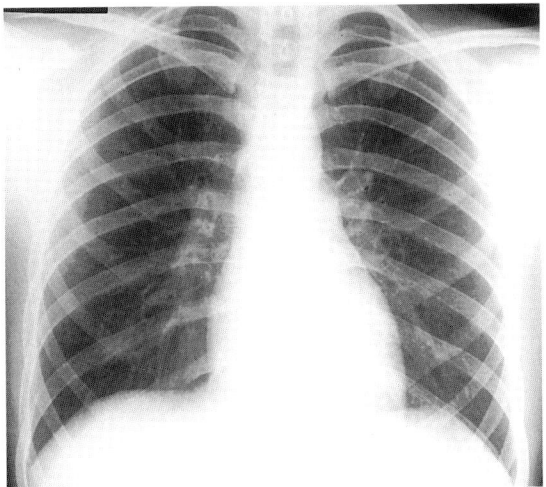

Fig. 27.2
Chest radiograph on admission. The cardiac silhouette is normal.

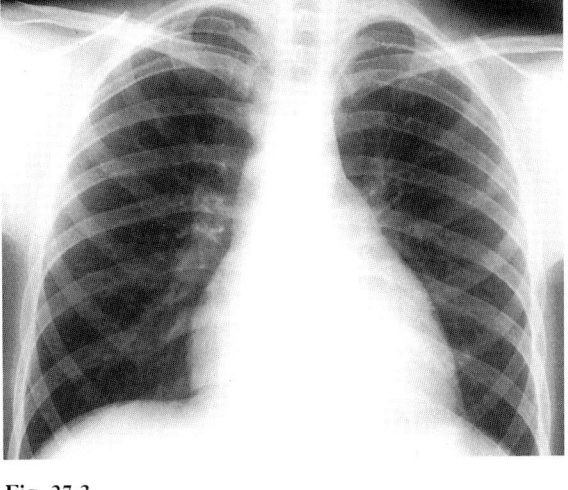

Fig. 27.3
Chest radiograph 5 days after admission. The cardiothoracic ratio is increased.

Additional investigations
An ECG showed characteristic abnormalities (Fig. 27.1). The chest radiograph on admission was normal (Fig. 27.2).

DIAGNOSIS
The history of sharp chest pain varying with posture and the presence of a pericardial rub are typical features of pericarditis. The diagnosis was confirmed by the characteristic ECG changes of ST elevation which is concave upwards. Chest pain following a 'viral' type illness in a young person usually indicates either pericardial or pleural inflammation. Influenza virus or Coxsackie virus are the pathogens commonly implicated.

OUTCOME
He was treated with bed rest and an oral NSAID. The pericardial friction rub was heard intermittently over the first 2 days of admission and then disappeared. The fever and pain subsided. Five days after admission a follow-up chest radiograph revealed apparent cardiac enlargement (Fig. 27.3). This appearance on the chest radiograph following pericarditis is suggestive of a pericardial effusion, and was confirmed by echocardiography (Fig. 27.4). Most effusions following viral pericarditis are small and not of haemodynamic significance. As he was asymptomatic he was discharged home with an outpatient review appointment 2 weeks later.

At the time of review he was well and a repeat chest radiograph revealed that the cardiac silhouette had returned to normal.

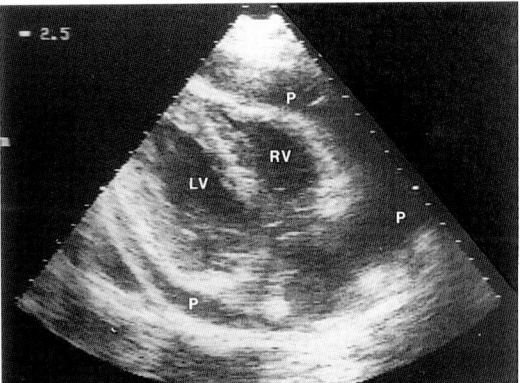

Fig. 27.4
Echocardiographic view (two-dimensional) showing pericardial effusion (P), left ventricle (LV) and right ventricle (RV).

KEY POINTS

History/Examination
- Pericardial pain is sharp and often varies with posture.
- Pericardial friction rubs are often transient.

Investigations
- ST elevation (concave upwards) on the ECG is typical of pericarditis.
- Echocardiography is the investigation of choice to show a pericardial effusion.

Outcome
- Viral pericarditis is usually a self-limiting illness.

28 Andrew Munro (19)
Breathlessness, abdominal pain

CASE HISTORY
Mr Munro was attending an employment training course and had spent the previous 2 weeks in a boarding house. He had been previously very healthy, but for the last few days had been unduly tired and had developed a sore throat. He had treated himself with aspirin, planning to contact his general practitioner if he felt no better when he returned home at the weekend. He had not eaten much during his illness but had been particularly thirsty, including during the night when he had also been rising to pass water. He tried to attend his classes but on the penultimate day had returned to his room early to go to bed. During the night he became progressively unwell and developed persistent central abdominal pain and nausea. His landlady, on missing him at breakfast the following morning, visited his room and found him still lying in bed. His breathing was laboured, he appeared drowsy and moaned as he held his hands to his abdomen. His landlady called an emergency ambulance and he was taken directly to hospital.

EXAMINATION
On admission he was flushed and had deep, sighing respiration. He made little attempt at spontaneous communication but gave appropriate responses to direct questioning. He was pyrexial at 37.7°C, his pulse was 130/min and blood pressure was 96/60. His mouth was dry, his fauces reddened and he had some palpable cervical lymph nodes. He had no neck stiffness and no added sounds on auscultation of the heart and lungs. He was lean and his abdomen was scaphoid and tense. Tenderness limited palpation, but there was no apparent organomegaly and bowel sounds were audible. There were no signs of focal neurological abnormality.

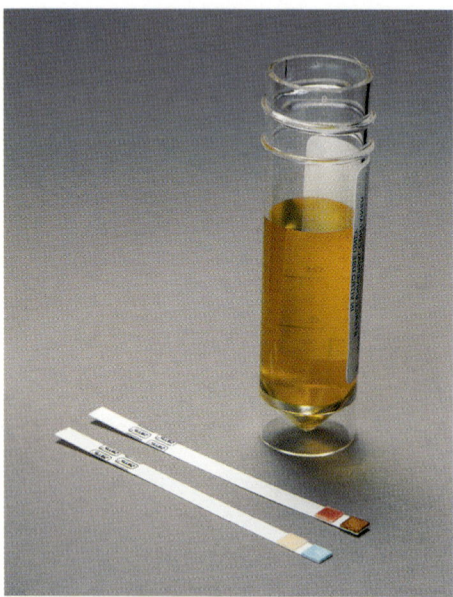

Fig. 28.1
Specimen of concentrated urine with test strip panels showing positive for glucose (brown) and ketones (purple); a control strip, which has been dipped in normal urine, is also shown for comparison.

INVESTIGATIONS
Routine investigation results

Urine	SpG 1.023	Pr neg	Glu ++++	Ke +++	Blood neg
Serum	Na 130	K 5.8	HCO_3 9	U 11.4	Cr 127
	Alb 35	Bil 18	AAT 19	AP 106	γGT 52
Blood	Hb 169	MCV 92	WCC 18.5	Plt 293	ESR 28

Additional investigations
Arterial blood gases were as follows:

pH	pO_2	pCO_2	$sHCO_3$
7.09	13.1	2.8	11

Plasma glucose was 29.3 mmol/l (reference range < 8.0) and serum amylase was 420 U/l (< 340). Chest and abdominal radiographs were normal. A throat swab showed normal oral flora, and there was no growth from blood and urine cultures.

DIAGNOSIS

This previously well young man had developed ketoacidosis as the presenting manifestation of insulin-dependent (type 1) diabetes mellitus. Polyuria and polydipsia were the most important clues in the history. Alternative causes of polyuria and polydipsia, such as diabetes insipidus, hypokalaemia or hypercalcaemia, were unlikely given this type of presentation in a young patient, and psychogenic polydipsia is not typically associated with nocturnal thirst and polyuria. Urinalysis by dipstick testing quickly confirmed the presence of glycosuria and ketonuria (Fig. 28.1); when a patient is too unwell to cooperate with providing urine, it is reasonable to consider bladder catheterization. Although the degree of acidosis can only be precisely measured by arterial blood gas analysis, a low venous bicarbonate level is a useful guide as to its severity. A viral upper respiratory infection may have precipitated his acute presentation, although his sore throat may merely have been a consequence of inadequate hydration. His apparent breathlessness was in fact Kussmaul respiration, the typical hyperventilatory response in an attempt to compensate for a metabolic acidosis. Diabetic ketoacidosis can also produce abdominal findings that closely mimic an acute surgical problem, as in this case. Slight elevation in serum amylase is a common, non-specific finding in an acutely unwell individual; the value was much too low in this case to support a diagnosis of acute pancreatitis.

OUTCOME

Following rehydration and infusion of insulin, with careful monitoring of serum potassium concentration, his clinical condition improved rapidly and his abdominal pain settled. A broad-spectrum antibiotic was given empirically but there was no definite evidence of any bacterial infection. A family history of type 1 diabetes or other organ-specific autoimmune disease is not unusual in such cases and, indeed, on his recovery, further enquiry revealed that his mother had been treated for thyroid disease and a maternal aunt was on insulin treatment. Mr Munro was established on subcutaneous insulin therapy, taught how to monitor his blood glucose and allowed home 4 days after admission.

KEY POINTS

History/Examination
- Ketoacidotic coma may be the initial presentation of diabetes mellitus.
- Consider diabetic ketoacidosis in the differential diagnosis of an ill patient presenting with an 'acute' abdomen.

Investigations
- Blood glucose should always be measured at the bedside in a patient with altered consciousness of unknown cause.
- The presence of ketonuria can be quickly demonstrated by a dipstick test.

Outcome
- Diabetic ketoacidosis is fatal if not detected and treated promptly.

29 John Reid (77) Right-sided weakness

CASE HISTORY

Mr Reid was a retired hospital porter. Two days before his admission he was talking on the telephone when he noticed some difficulty with his speech, particularly in finding names for some objects. Later that day he became unsteady while walking and felt that his right leg had become weak. During the next few hours the difficulty in walking became more severe such that he fell. He struck the side of his head on a coffee table and was unable to rise thereafter. He managed to summon help from his neighbour who brought him to hospital. On admission, the neighbour mentioned that Mr Reid had suffered some headaches affecting the back of his head and neck during the past 2 weeks. These had occurred while he was sitting reading and Mr Reid had attributed them to bad posture.

He had been hypertensive for 7 years and was treated with a thiazide diuretic. He smoked 10 cigarettes per day and drank five pints of beer each week. He lived alone in a first floor apartment, and prior to this illness had been able to live independently.

EXAMINATION

He was alert and orientated, but had difficulty in giving a history, with particular problems in naming people and objects. He was apyrexial. His pulse was 80/min and regular, and blood pressure was 150/100. The carotid pulses were palpable and there were no carotid bruits. His heart sounds were normal with no added sounds. Chest and abdominal examination was negative, and there was no neck stiffness. He had right-sided facial weakness (Fig. 29.1a); however, this did not affect the upper part of the face or eye closure (Fig. 29.1b). Cranial nerves were otherwise intact. Power was decreased in the right arm and absent in the right leg; reflexes were reduced in the right arm and leg. The right plantar response was extensor.

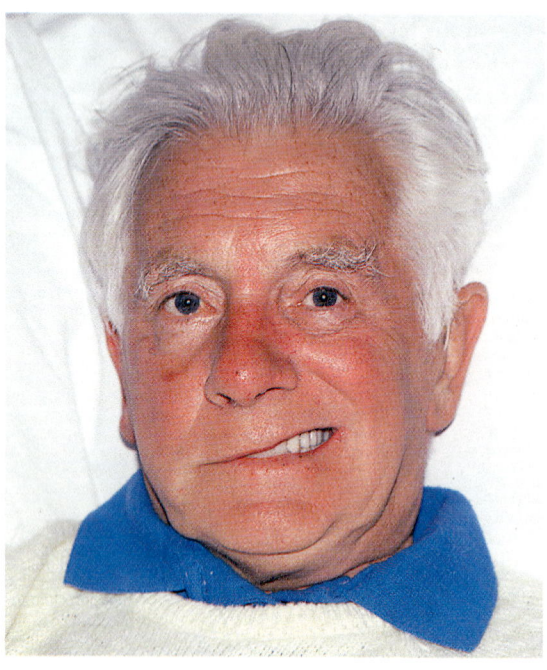

(a)

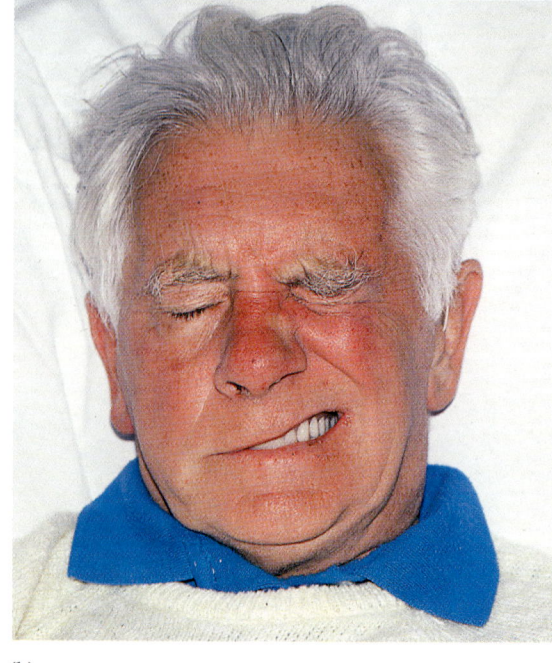

(b)

Fig. 29.1
Facial view showing (a) paralysis of the lower right face and (b) preservation of eye closure.

INVESTIGATIONS
Routine investigation results

Urine	SpG 1025	Pr neg	Glu neg	Ke tr	Blood neg
Serum	Na 140	K 4.7	HCO3 25	U 6.0	Cr 101
	Alb 45	Bil 7	AAT 22	AP 71	γGT 31
Blood	Hb 132	MCV 95	WCC 7.2	Plt 337	ESR 25

Additional investigations
The CT head scan is shown in Fig. 29.2.

DIAGNOSIS
The right facial weakness with sparing of the muscles of the upper face is a sign of an upper motor neurone lesion. The speech difficulty is dysphasia. The clinical signs of upper motor neurone facial weakness together with weakness in the right arm and leg and dysphasia suggest that the abnormality is in the territory of the left middle cerebral artery. The CT scan confirms infarction in this area together with diffuse ischaemic change throughout the remainder of the brain. The history suggests that the infarction has evolved gradually, which is less common than a sudden onset of neurological deficit (acute completed stroke). The headaches are probably incidental and unrelated to the infarction, although headache may be a prominent symptom in patients in whom a cerebral haemorrhage has occurred.

Cerebral infarction may be due to vascular thrombosis close to the site of infarction, embolization of material from atheromatous plaques in the arterial system (e.g. internal carotid artery) or embolization of thrombi from more distant sources (e.g. the heart, following myocardial infarction or arrhythmia). The absence of a carotid bruit does not exclude significant atheroma in the internal carotid system. Risk factors for cerebrovascular disease in this patient included hypertension and smoking.

The diagnosis of cerebrovascular accident can often be made clinically. Reflexes are often decreased immediately after a cerebrovascular accident, subsequently becoming increased with or without clonus. A CT scan was indicated in this case to exclude other space-occupying lesions such as tumour or subdural haematoma which might be associated with gradual onset of symptoms and headache, and to assess whether the lesion was an infarct or haemorrhage.

OUTCOME
Mr Reid underwent physiotherapy, speech therapy and occupational therapy, and during the following 3 months made a partial functional recovery. Some return of power occurred in the right leg although he remained unable to walk unaided. Finger flexion and grip strength improved in the right hand but power remained substantially reduced in the right arm. Once the CT scan had confirmed the lesion to be a cerebral infarction, he was treated with low-dose aspirin to reduce the risk of recurrent infarction. He was advised to stop smoking. He was subsequently unable to return to independent existence, and required long-term care in a nursing home.

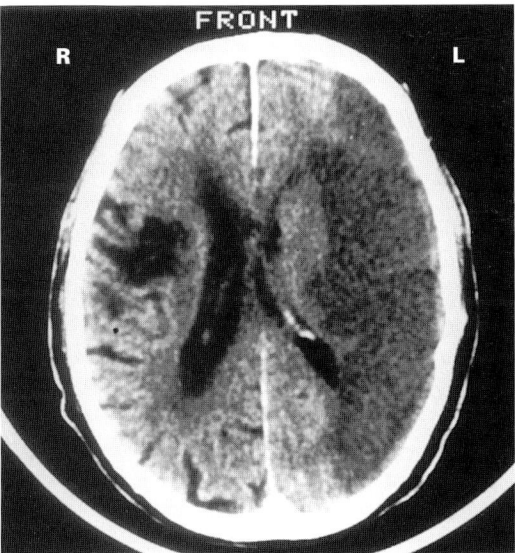

Fig. 29.2
A single transverse CT section through the head at the level of the lateral ventricles showing extensive infarction in the left middle cerebral artery territory.

KEY POINTS

History/Examination
- Stroke is typically, but not always, completed within a few hours.
- The site of a cerebral infarction or haemorrhage may be inferred from the pattern of neurological deficit.

Investigations
- CT scanning is useful to confirm the diagnosis and to plan appropriate therapy.

Outcome
- Social circumstances are important in determining outcome.

George Dunn (68)
Sweats, weight loss

CASE HISTORY
Mr Dunn, a retired farmer with a 10-year history of emphysema, complained to his general practitioner of increasing shortness of breath and a cough productive of purulent sputum. This was initially thought to be an exacerbation of his chronic obstructive lung disease and he was therefore commenced on a course of oral prednisolone and amoxycillin. Despite this, he failed to improve and 6 weeks later he was admitted to hospital with increasing breathlessness, intermittent sweats and weight loss of 6 kg.

He recollected having had a chest radiograph (Fig. 30.1) 6 years previously when he had a 'chest infection'. On that occasion, he was told he had a 'shadow' in the right lung, but that it did not require any specific treatment.

He was a widower who lived on a farm dealing mainly with livestock. For many years after the death of his wife he had also had a part-time job as a barman. He had smoked heavily for 40 years and admitted to drinking only a moderate amount of alcohol.

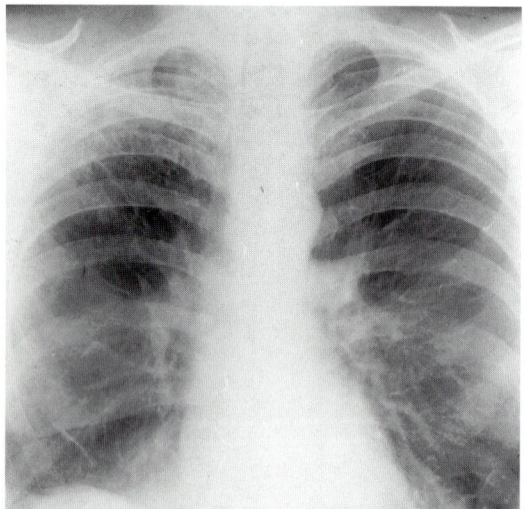

Fig. 30.1
Chest radiograph showing streaky opacification in the right upper zone.

EXAMINATION
He was thin and looked unwell with central cyanosis and a fever (37.8°C). He had enlarged non-tender cervical lymph nodes. His pulse was 110/min and regular, and blood pressure was 110/60. Respiratory examination revealed hyperinflation of the chest with dullness to percussion and coarse crackles over the left lung apex. A few rhonchi were audible over the right lung. The liver edge was palpable 1 cm below the costal margin but the remainder of the examination was normal.

INVESTIGATIONS
Routine investigation results

Urine	SpG 1.005	Pr neg	Glu neg	Ke neg	Blood neg
Serum	Na 135	K 3.7	HCO_3 26	U 3.1	Cr 88
	Alb 35	Bil 14	AAT 35	AP 123	γGT 134
Blood	Hb 132	MCV 100	WCC 4.5	Plt 345	ESR 81

Additional investigations
The blood film showed round macrocytes and stomatocytes. Arterial blood gases (breathing air) were as follows:

pH	pO_2	pCO_2	$sHCO_3$
7.35	7.5	3.4	26

Blood cultures were sterile after 48 h incubation. The chest radiograph (Fig. 30.2) showed changes from the previous one. Sputum microscopy provided the diagnosis (Fig. 30.3).

DIAGNOSIS
Gradual onset of fever, night sweats, malaise and cough are typical of tuberculosis, and the history of a previous 'shadow' on the chest radiograph raises the possibility of reactivation of previous tuberculous infection. This was confirmed in Mr Dunn's case

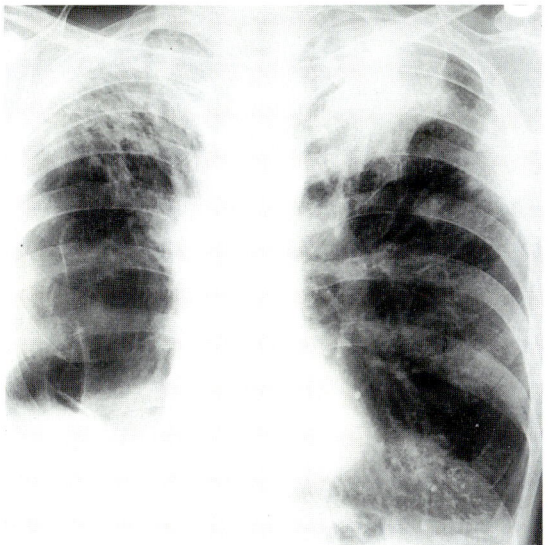

Fig. 30.2
Chest radiograph showing opacification in both upper zones with cavitation on the left.

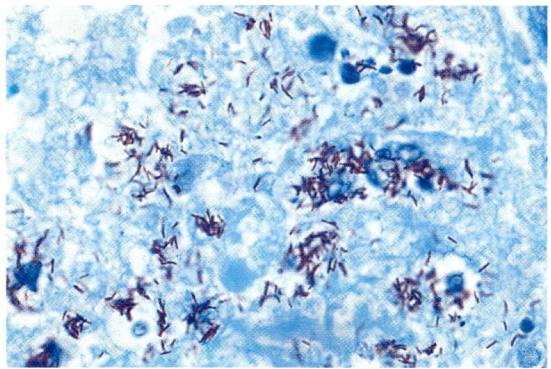

Fig. 30.3
Ziehl-Neelsen stain of sputum smear showing numerous acid and alcohol-fast bacilli.

by sputum microscopy, which showed acid and alcohol-fast bacilli and the subsequent growth of *Mycobacterium tuberculosis* on culture of the sputum.

The shadowing noted in the apex of the right lung in the earlier chest radiograph (Fig. 30.1) was typical of fibrosis related to previous tuberculosis. The current admission chest radiograph (Fig. 30.2) shows bilateral upper zone opacities with cavitation in the left upper lobe related to the current infection.

The blood film appearances and the abnormal liver enzymes are suggestive of chronic alcohol excess, which, together with the recent course of steroid that he had received, are risk factors for reactivation of tuberculosis.

OUTCOME
Mr Dunn was treated with rifampicin, isoniazid and pyrazinamide (triple antituberculous therapy) for 8 weeks. After this time, culture results confirmed the growth of *M. tuberculosis* sensitive to all of these agents. Pyrazinamide was stopped and he continued isoniazid and rifampicin for a further 4 months. The steroids were withdrawn gradually over a 2-week period. All close contacts were screened for tuberculosis.

KEY POINTS
History/Examination
- Tuberculosis is an important cause of respiratory infection.
- Abnormal physical signs in the chest are often minimal in tuberculosis.

Investigations
- Sputum should be stained for acid and alcohol-fast bacilli.
- Mycobacterial culture is necessary to identify the specific organism.

Outcome
- Antibiotic sensitivity testing of *Mycobacteria* is a useful guide to therapy.
- Notification of tuberculosis cases is mandatory in the UK to permit screening of contacts.

Catherine Glass (76) 'Off Her Legs'

CASE HISTORY

Mrs Glass, a widow, had been just about coping at home on her own with the support of a home help twice per week, and a married daughter who visited most days. She had not been in good health for some years and suffered from chronic obstructive airways disease and congestive cardiac failure, both of which were aggravated by her considerable obesity. She was on long-term treatment with a bronchodilator inhaler and diuretics; the diuretic dose had been increased twice in the previous 6 months on account of her exertional dyspnoea. There had always been some doubt as to her compliance with the prescribed therapy.

Three weeks earlier she had been admitted as an emergency with vomiting and abdominal pain thought to be due to strangulation of a femoral hernia. At that stage her urea, electrolytes and creatinine were near normal and she proceeded to successful reduction of the hernia under spinal anaesthesia. She made a good initial recovery but was unsteady on her feet, and so after a week she was transferred to a nursing home as a temporary resident for a fortnight's convalescence. Her progress continued to be disappointing and towards the end of her stay she was too unsteady on her feet to stand or attempt to walk, preferring to lie in bed all day. She was clearly unable to return home and was admitted to the receiving medical ward for assessment. She described general lethargy and weakness in her limbs, poor appetite and dizziness on standing. She was, as usual, breathless on minor exertion but had no cough, sputum or chest pain. There was no recent history of headache, visual or auditory failure, and no peripheral sensory disturbance.

Past medical history included cholecystectomy at age 36 years, hysterectomy at age 48 years and hiatus hernia demonstrated on barium meal at age 60 years. There was no family history of note. Mrs Glass's current medication consisted of frusemide 80 mg twice daily, amiloride 5 mg daily, ranitidine 150 mg at night, temazepam 10 mg at night and salbutamol by inhaler.

EXAMINATION

On admission she was quiet and rather withdrawn. She was grossly obese. There was no fever, pallor, cyanosis or abnormal pigmentation. She was dyspnoeic on minor exertion and had scattered crackles and wheezes on auscultation of the chest. Her pulse was 84/min and regular; her blood pressure was 122/78 in the right arm supine, and 96/66 on standing, whereupon she had to be supported by two nurses. The jugular venous pulse was not visible and there was no peripheral oedema. There was no apparent organomegaly in her large abdomen; the hernia scar was healing well. There were no focal neurological signs but she was unable to maintain an upright posture. Fundoscopy was normal.

INVESTIGATIONS
Routine investigation results

Urine	SpG 1.019	Pr tr	Glu neg	Ke neg	Blood neg
Serum	Na 127	K 5.5	HCO_3 20	U 19.3	Cr 233
	Alb 33	Bil 14	AAT 18	AP 104	γGT 29
Blood	Hb 120	MCV 82	WCC 5.8	Plt 216	ESR 19

Additional investigations

A chest radiograph showed slight cardiomegaly and some hyperinflation of the lungs but no focal pulmonary abnormality. An ECG showed sinus rhythm and no diagnostic abnormalities.

Random plasma glucose was 7.2 mmol/l (reference range < 8.0), serum osmolality 294 mOsm/kg (278–305) and urine osmolality 556 mOsm/kg (350–1000). Urinary sodium excretion was 41 mmol/24h (100–250 mmol/24h on normal diet). A short Synacthen test showed basal plasma cortisol at 9 am was 394 nmol/l (230–620); 30 min after an intramuscular injection of soluble tetracosactrin (0.25 mg) it rose to 681 nmol/l (normal increment > 200).

DIAGNOSIS

The patient was suffering from the effects of overenthusiastic diuretic therapy resulting in salt depletion, reduced intravascular volume and renal hypoperfusion with impaired renal function. The development of symptomatic postural hypotension is an important clue. A low serum sodium and continued excretion of urinary sodium at a subnormal, yet inappropriately high, rate (in the face of hyponatraemia) confirmed a renal salt-losing state. The normal osmolality excluded the syndrome of inappropriate antidiuretic hormone release (SIADH) as a cause of the hyponatraemia and the short Synacthen test excluded adrenocortical insufficiency. The rising serum potassium concentration was due to a combination of renal impairment and administration of a potassium-sparing diuretic (amiloride), and could have reached a potentially life-threatening level if unchecked.

The reason for the sudden deterioration in this patient's condition, despite there being no immediate change in her regular medication, relates to the issue of drug compliance. Her initial diuretic prescription for left ventricular failure was appropriate and beneficial; the decision to increase the dose in the face of recurrent features of cardiac failure was inappropriate as it did not take account of the fact she had not been taking the prescribed dose regularly. Poor compliance protected her from the effects of diuretic overtreatment until she went into hospital for hernia repair whereupon her medication was administered as prescribed and she quickly developed the diuretic-related problems described.

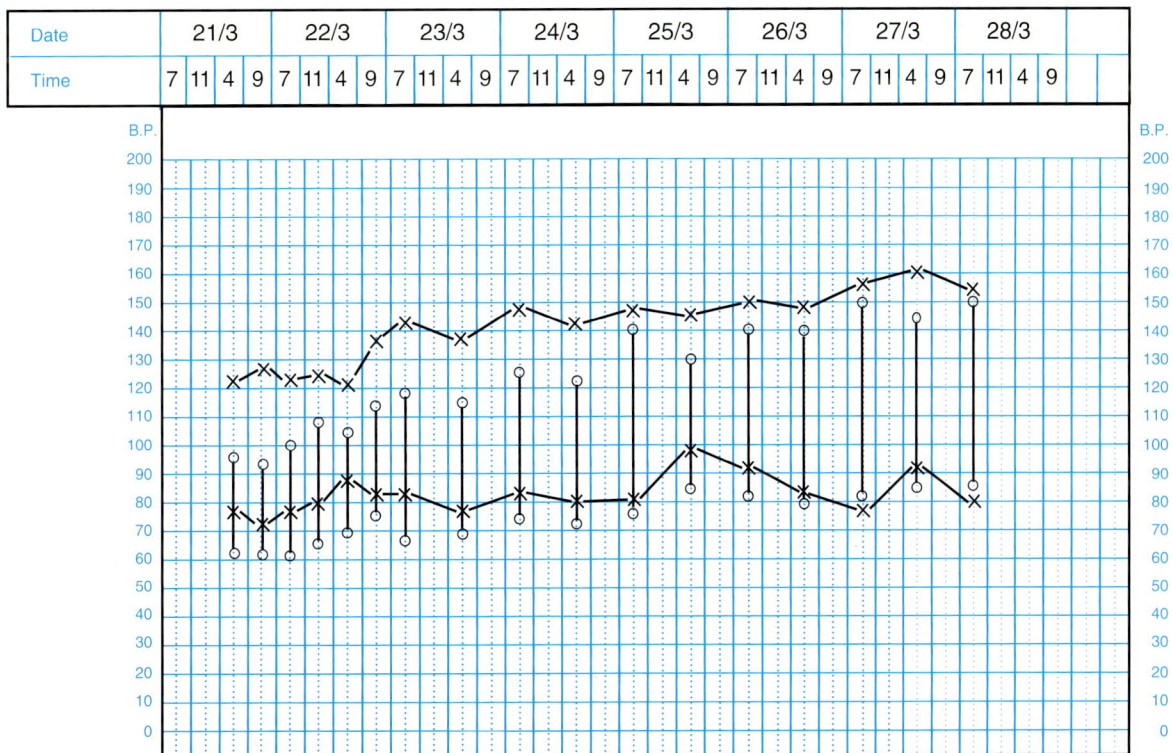

Fig. 31.1
Erect and supine blood pressure chart showing initial postural hypotension resolving with reduction in diuretic therapy.

OUTCOME

The diuretic therapy was stopped for several days during which the postural hypotension resolved (Fig. 31.1), and the patient's general condition and mobility improved markedly. Renal function improved to a level similar to that recorded on her admission for surgery (creatinine 124 μmol/l) and the electrolyte levels returned to normal. She was discharged home to resume her largely independent existence 4 weeks later on 40 mg frusemide daily. This patient's recovery from severe functional impairment and multiple biochemical abnormalities was entirely dependent on recognition of her medication-related problem and simply stopping the excessive diuretic treatment.

KEY POINTS

History/Examination
- Iatrogenic (doctor-induced) disease is very common.
- Consider whether problems with compliance are affecting the response to prescribed medication.
- Measurement of erect and supine blood pressure is essential in patients who complain of dizziness.

Investigations
- Hyponatraemia associated with continued urinary sodium loss and normal serum osmolality indicates inappropriate renal salt loss.

Outcome
- Withdrawal of inappropriate medication can sometimes produce dramatic clinical improvement.

Derek Southcote (23)
Swollen neck

CASE HISTORY

Mr Southcote, a graphic designer, had recently returned home to the countryside, after completing a 6-month contract in London. For about 3 weeks prior to leaving London, he had complained of tiredness and weakness, and had noticed that he was sweating excessively at night. He had also had some dull, aching central chest discomfort, which was continuous and unrelated to meals or activity. The pain was partially relieved by analgesics. For 2 weeks prior to attending the clinic, he had noted swelling in the right side of his neck such that he was having difficulty in fastening his collar. The swelling was not painful, but appeared to be progressively increasing in size. His appetite had been rather poor and he had lost about 5 kg in weight, but he had no other specific symptoms.

He denied any significant previous medical illnesses apart from chickenpox in childhood. He was not on medication and was a non-smoker. He had used marihuana occasionally in the past, and had a brief homosexual relationship at the age of 18 years. He was currently living alone in a small cottage. There was no family history of note.

EXAMINATION

He looked pale and generally unwell, with some scratch marks on both forearms. There was a large, firm swelling in the right side of the neck, which was not tender. He had an intermittent fever (Fig. 32.1). Careful examination also revealed some small palpable lymph nodes in the groins bilaterally. His pulse rate was 76/min and regular, and blood pressure was 110/75. His heart sounds were normal and there were no signs of cardiac failure. His chest was clinically normal. His liver was palpable 1 cm below the costal margin and his spleen was enlarged to 3 cm below the costal margin. There were no other palpable abdominal masses, bowel sounds were normal and rectal examination was normal. There were no focal neurological abnormalities.

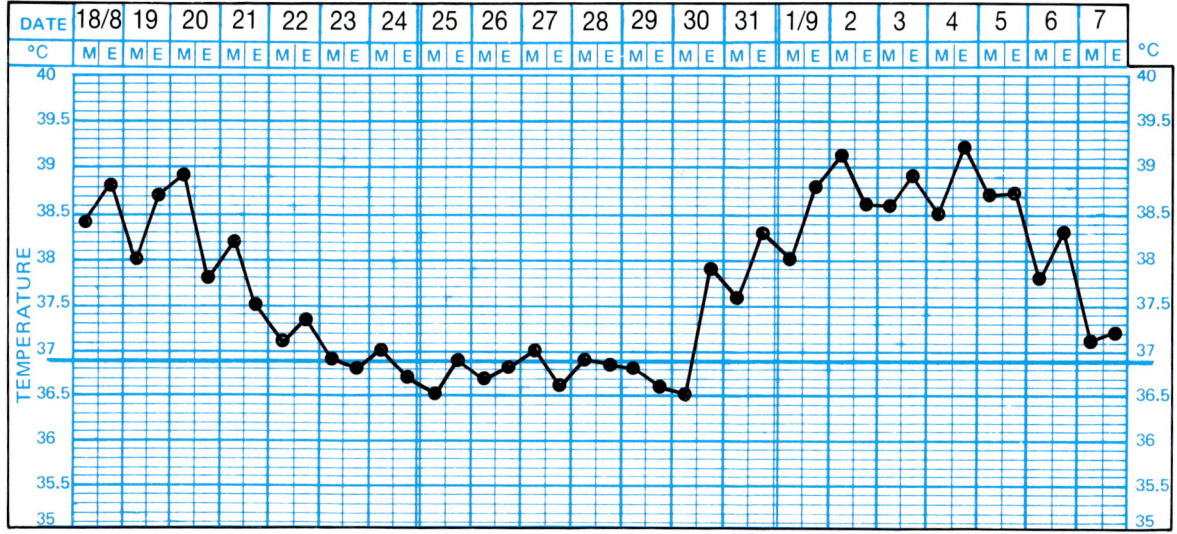

Fig. 32.1
Temperature chart showing intermittent fever (Pel-Ebstein fever).

INVESTIGATIONS
Routine investigation results

Urine	SpG 1015	Pr neg	Glu neg	Ke neg	Blood neg
Serum	Na 136	K 4.2	HCO$_3$ 24	U 6.0	Cr 95
	Alb 37	Bil 6	AAT 42	AP 112	γGT 47
Blood	Hb 95	MCV 90	WCC 12.6	Plt 522	ESR 42

Additional investigations

The differential white cell count was normal. An HIV test, carried out with informed consent, was negative. Serum uric acid was 0.37 mmol/l (reference range < 0.42).

The chest radiograph (Fig. 32.2) showed evidence of mediastinal lymphadenopathy. An abdominal CT scan confirmed that the liver and spleen were enlarged with evidence of infiltration by tumour and, in addition, revealed evidence of retroperitoneal lymph node enlargement. Bone marrow appearances were normal. A biopsy was taken of the mass in his neck (Fig. 32.3).

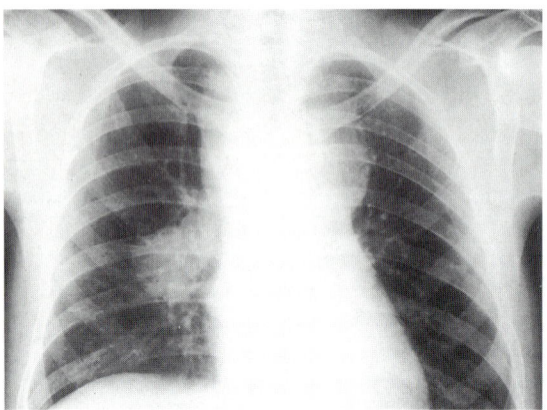

Fig. 32.2
Chest radiograph showing mediastinal and right hilar lymphadenopathy.

DIAGNOSIS

In a young person with lymphadenopathy and a history of constitutional symptoms such as fever and malaise, lymphoma must be considered as a likely diagnosis. The associated findings of hepatosplenomegaly and abdominal lymph node enlargement in this case are also suggestive of lymphoma. Lymph node biopsy provided the most rapid method of establishing the diagnosis and the pathological features (Fig. 32.3) were diagnostic of Hodgkin's lymphoma.

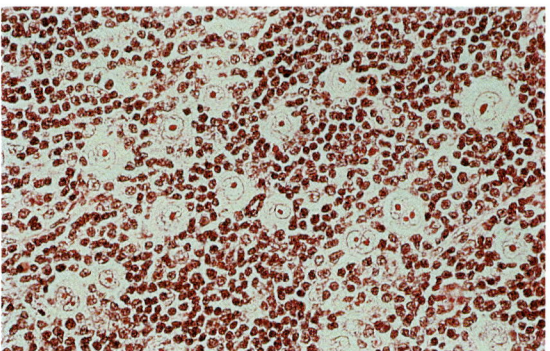

Fig. 32.3
Lymph node biopsy showing replacement of normal node architecture by an infiltrate of lymphoid cells, including many Hodgkin's and Reed-Sternberg cells.

Clinical staging of the disease by CT scan to define the groups of affected lymph nodes and the involvement of other organs (such as spleen and liver) was important as a guide to appropriate therapy, as was bone marrow examination with immunophenotyping of cells to assess marrow involvement. In Mr Southcote's case, widespread involvement of lymph nodes associated with the presence of constitutional symptoms such as intermittent fever and sweats indicated that systemic chemotherapy was necessary.

Alternative diagnoses considered before obtaining the diagnostic biopsy included toxoplasmosis, Epstein Barr virus infection, HIV infection, and tuberculosis.

OUTCOME

He was treated with combination chemotherapy and was given allopurinol to prevent drug-induced gout. His lymphadenopathy and systemic symptoms resolved and the clinical and CT appearances of the liver and spleen improved over the next 5 months. Eleven months after presentation he had a further relapse.

KEY POINTS

History/Examination
- The combination of malaise, night sweats and weight loss is suggestive of lymphoma.
- Palpation of all lymph node groups is important in such patients.

Investigations
- Lymph node biopsy allows a histological diagnosis.
- Whole-body CT scanning and bone marrow biopsy are used to determine the extent of lymphoma.

Outcome
- The choice of treatment for lymphoma is dictated by clinical and pathological staging.

Janette Barton (15) Headache
33

CASE HISTORY

Miss Barton, who attended a local boarding school, went to the school warden complaining of tiredness and an unproductive cough that had been present for about 2 days. The warden thought she might have 'flu, gave her some paracetamol and advised her to rest in bed. The following day she was no better and complained of feeling hot and sweaty, with an increasing headache despite taking paracetamol. Her eyes had become uncomfortable when in bright light and she had noticed a rash over her arms and legs, which was spreading to her trunk.

She had previously been well except for mild asthma for which she used a salbutamol inhaler. She had been a boarder at this school for 4 years and the two girls with whom she shared a room had not been unwell.

EXAMINATION

On admission she was febrile (38.2°C) and distressed with headache but was lucid and able to give a history. Discrete petechial lesions were present over the arms, legs and shoulders (Fig. 33.1). There was marked neck stiffness and Kernig's sign was positive. Her optic fundi were normal and there were no focal neurological abnormalities. Her pulse was 120/min and regular, and blood pressure was 110/50. Her chest was clear and abdominal examination was normal.

INVESTIGATIONS
Routine investigation results

Urine	SpG 1.012	Pr neg	Glu neg	Ke +	Blood neg
Serum	Na 129	K 4.0	HCO₃ 17	U 3.4	Cr 78
	Alb 35	Bil 20	AAT 30	AP 150	γGT 23
Blood	Hb 130	MCV 87	WCC 18.7	Plt 200	ESR 45

Additional investigations

A differential white blood cell count revealed a neutrophil leucocytosis. Blood cultures were sterile and a throat swab was negative. Blood glucose was 10 mmol/l (reference range < 8).

A lumbar puncture was performed, and showed cloudy CSF with a pressure of 23 cm. The fluid contained 1280 white cells/mm^3 of which 70% were polymorphs and 30% lymphocytes. The protein level was 876 g/l and glucose was 4.0 mmol/l (40% of blood glucose). The Gram stain of the CSF is shown in Fig. 33.2. Blood and CSF latex agglutination tests were positive for meningococcal antigen.

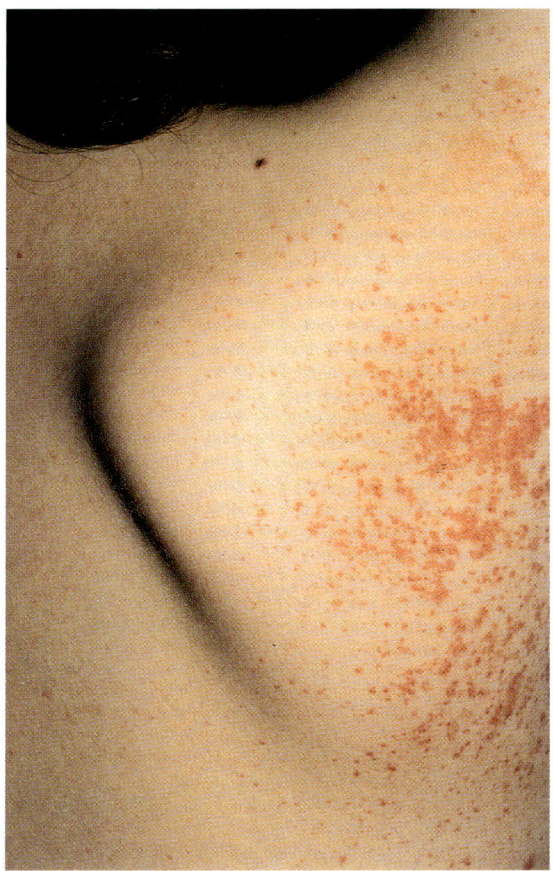

Fig. 33.1
Petechial rash overlying the scapula.

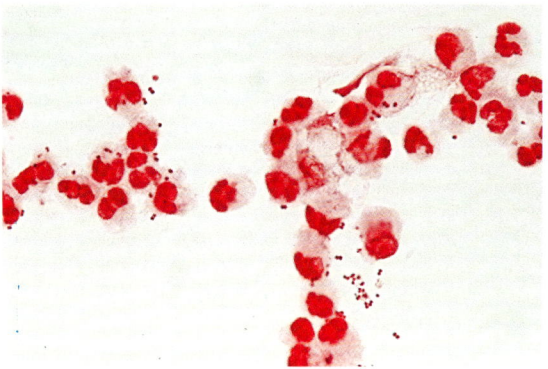

Fig. 33.2
Gram stain of cerebrospinal fluid showing polymorphonuclear leucocytes and Gram-negative diplococci, some of which are intracellular.

DIAGNOSIS

The history of headache, fever, lethargy and stiff neck is typical of meningitis, and the presence of a petechial rash strongly suggests meningococcal infection. The diagnosis was confirmed by the finding of turbid CSF containing a high white cell count with Gram-negative diplococci and a positive latex agglutination test. Peripheral neutrophil leucocytosis is a common feature of meningococcal meningitis. The onset of the illness in this patient was subacute over 3 days, but is more often acute, and death may occur within a few hours. Lumbar puncture should therefore be performed urgently unless increased intracranial pressure is suspected, in which case a CT scan of the head should be performed to show the presence of cerebral oedema or a cerebral abscess. Increased intracranial pressure is suggested clinically by the presence of papilloedema or focal neurological abnormalities.

OUTCOME

She was treated with high doses of intravenous benzylpenicillin for 7 days, and made a complete recovery. Her room-mates were given a course of prophylactic oral rifampicin. Miss Barton was also given rifampicin at the time of discharge to eradicate nasopharyngeal carriage of the meningococcus.

KEY POINTS

History/Examination
- Neck stiffness, headache and fever are the typical features of meningococcal meningitis.
- Impaired consciousness is a bad prognostic sign in meningitis.

Investigations
- Urgent investigation of suspected meningitis is necessary.
- CSF examination is the most important investigation in the diagnosis of meningitis.

Outcome
- Bacterial meningitis requires urgent treatment with intravenous antibiotics in high doses.
- Prophylaxis with rifampicin is indicated for close contacts (e.g household contacts, room-mates) of the index case.

Walter Gilbert (81) Breathlessness

CASE HISTORY
Mr Gilbert was referred to the medical outpatient clinic with a few months' history of poor appetite and occasional vomiting. He was unsure if there had been any weight loss, but with the accompanying deterioration in his general health, his general practitioner had been wondering whether there may be an underlying malignancy. It was noted in the referral letter that part of the problem may be a psychological reaction to his wife's recent death from breast cancer; Mr Gilbert had temporarily moved in with his son and daughter-in-law. At the clinic, he denied most symptoms but did admit to being breathless on exertion with occasional chest 'tightness', and having intermittent vague abdominal discomfort. He appeared frail and a little pale. He refused admission for investigation, agreeing only to attend as an outpatient for a barium meal examination.

A week later, he was admitted as an emergency with worsening of his breathlessness, which was now present at rest. There had been no change in his nausea and vomiting, he had no difficulty in swallowing and there was no alteration of bowel habit. He denied having any cough or sputum and gave no history of any urinary or neurological symptoms.

Past medical history included an inguinal hernia repair in his fifties, and a myocardial infarction at age 75 years. Mr Gilbert was a retired clerk. He had stopped smoking after his myocardial infarction, and his only medication was glyceryl trinitrate which he used, on average, three times per week.

EXAMINATION
On admission, Mr Gilbert was breathless at rest, and unable to lie flat. He was pale and apyrexial, and had a corneal arcus senilis (Fig. 34.1). There was a trace of ankle swelling. His jugular venous pulse was visible 8 cm above the sternal angle when he lay at 45°. His pulse was 96/min and regular, and blood pressure was 172/90. The heart sounds were normal and there were some fine, late inspiratory crepitations at both lung bases. The liver edge was smooth and palpable 2 cm below the costal margin, and there was a fullness below the umbilicus which was dull to percussion. Rectal examination revealed a large, smooth prostate gland. Faecal occult blood testing was negative. There were no abnormal neurological findings.

INVESTIGATIONS
Routine investigation results

Urine	SpG 1.015	Pr tr	Glu neg	Ke neg	Blood neg
Serum	Na 141	K 4.4	HCO$_3$ 18	U 16.9	Cr 310
	Alb 38	Bil 17	AAT 34	AP 117	γGT 58
Blood	Hb 100	MCV 84	WCC 9.4	Plt 321	ESR 17

Additional investigations
Serum cholesterol was 6.1 mmol/l (reference range 4.0–7.2) and prostate-specific antigen was 5.3 µg/l (< 10). A chest radiograph showed cardiomegaly and pulmonary oedema (Fig. 34.2). An ECG showed Q waves in the anterior leads signifying an old myocardial infarction and T wave inversion in the antero-lateral leads indicating ischaemia (Fig. 34.3). An abdominal ultrasound scan showed bilateral hydronephrosis and distension of the bladder with prominent trabeculation. (Fig. 34.4).

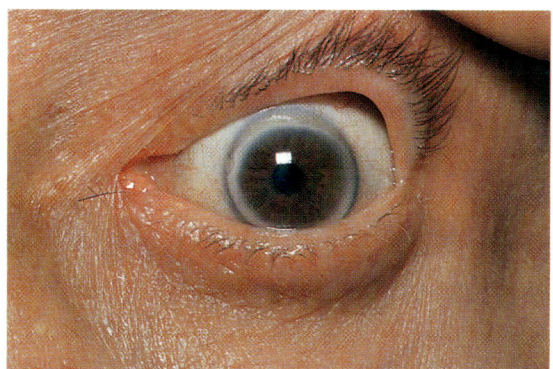

Fig. 34.1
Corneal arcus senilis.

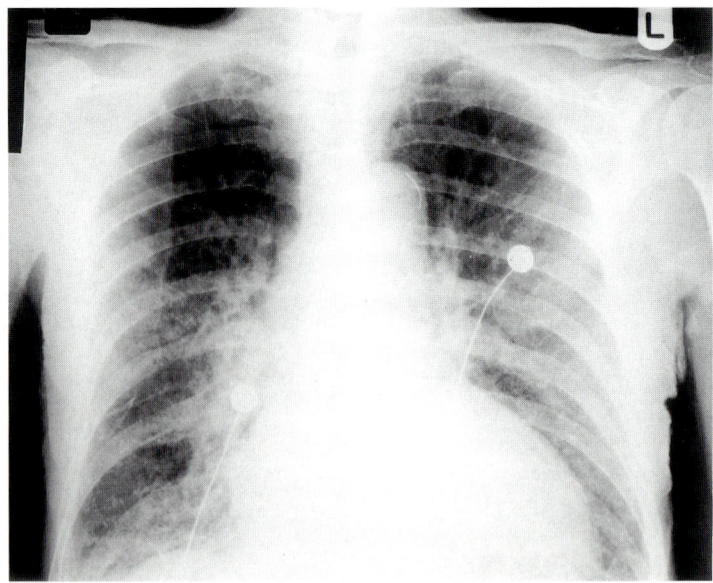

Fig. 34.2
Antero-posterior chest radiograph showing cardiomegaly, pulmonary oedema and electrocardiograph leads. Mural calcification is seen in the aortic arch.

DIAGNOSIS

This man had congestive cardiac failure associated with long-standing ischaemic heart disease and previous myocardial infarction. There was no evidence of acute myocardial infarction or paroxysmal dysrhythmia, but his cardiac failure had been exacerbated by fluid overload as a result of chronic renal failure due to bladder outlet obstruction. This had also been of some considerable duration as witnessed by the dilatation of the renal tract and hypertrophy of the bladder. The smooth feel of the prostate gland on rectal examination, and the normal level of prostate-specific antigen made prostatic malignancy unlikely. The normocytic anaemia was consequent upon chronic renal impairment. The abnormal liver function tests reflected hepatic congestion secondary to congestive cardiac failure.

Urinary frequency, including nocturia, hesitancy of micturition, poor urinary stream and dribbling

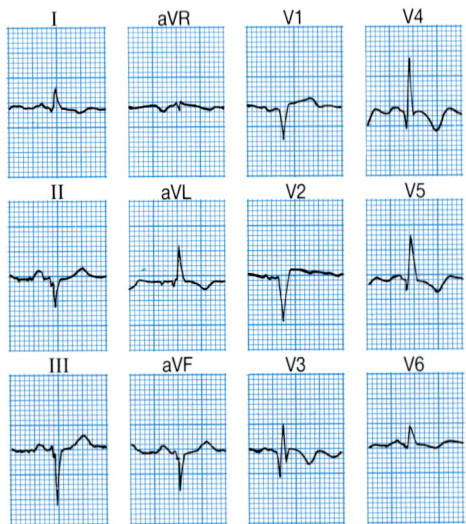

Fig. 34.3
ECG showing Q waves in leads V1–V5 indicating a previous full-thickness anterior myocardial infarction, and T wave inversion in I, aVL, and V3–V6 indicating lateral ischaemia.

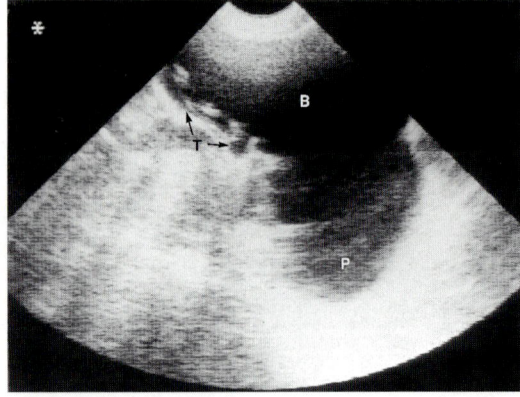

Fig. 34.4
Sagittal ultrasound scan section of the lower abdomen showing a distended urinary bladder (B) with a trabeculated wall (T) and an enlarged, smooth prostate gland (P).

incontinence, are typical symptoms of prostatism, but such a history is not always obtained. Detailed questioning of this patient, in the light of the diagnosis, still failed to reveal prostatic symptoms apart from some hesitancy of micturition.

While the presence of a corneal arcus suggests hyperlipidaemia in a younger patient, it is a common incidental finding in the elderly; the serum cholesterol in this man was unremarkable.

OUTCOME

A bladder catheter was inserted and 1600 ml of urine released over an hour. Mr Gilbert continued to have a good diuresis over the next 2–3 days without requiring diuretic therapy. His heart rate settled, his exercise tolerance improved and the lateral T wave changes on the ECG became less marked. After a month with an in-dwelling catheter his renal function had improved (creatinine 218 μmol/l; Hb 118 g/l) and his liver function tests returned to normal. He proceeded to transurethral resection of the prostate and histology confirmed benign prostatic hypertrophy.

KEY POINTS

History/Examination
- Bladder outlet obstruction may cause severe renal damage without reported symptoms of prostatism.
- Consider cardiac failure as a cause of hepatomegaly.
- Corneal arcus is a common incidental finding in the elderly.

Investigations
- Urinalysis may be normal in the presence of major urinary tract pathology.
- Ultrasound scanning is an ideal investigation for demonstrating the anatomy of the kidneys and bladder.
- Normocytic anaemia is a feature of chronic renal failure.

Outcome
- Relief of chronic bladder outlet obstruction can result in improvement in renal function.

Adam Currie (29)
Chest pain, breathlessness

CASE HISTORY

Mr Currie attended the hospital Emergency Department in the late afternoon in a distressed state, complaining of chest pain and increasing breathlessness. He had been walking his dog in the early morning when he suddenly developed a sharp pain in the right upper chest. After a few minutes, the pain lessened but was still present on coughing and he was unable to take a deep breath. He subsequently noticed breathlessness, which became increasingly severe as the day progressed. He had been able to go to his work as an accounts clerk, but during the afternoon he had become breathless at rest, and persuaded a friend to take him to hospital. The pain had decreased in intensity, although he was still aware of aching discomfort in the right chest.

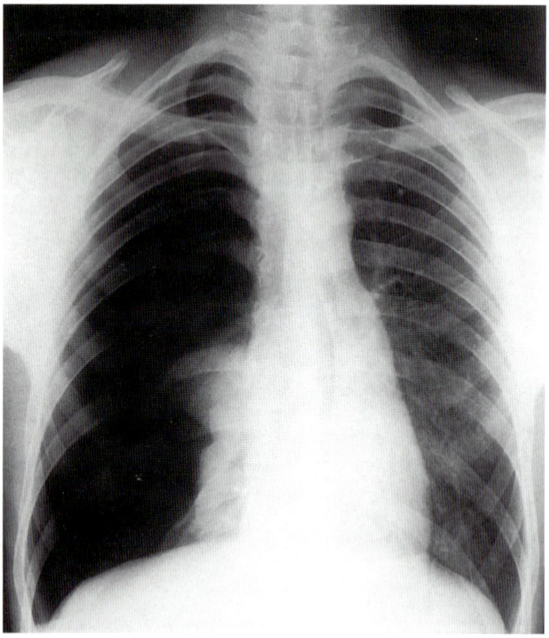

He had had an episode of left lower lobe pneumonia 5 years previously, when he had noticed chest pain of similar character, but had no other significant medical history. He was a non-smoker, drank a moderate amount of alcohol, and was a regular badminton player.

EXAMINATION

He was tall and thin and was distressed with breathlessness. His respiration was rapid (40/min) and shallow. On palpation, the trachea was deviated to the left, and percussion of the chest was resonant bilaterally. Breath sounds and vocal resonance were diminished over the right chest. His pulse rate was 130/min and regular, and blood pressure was 120/90. The cardiac apex beat was palpable in the anterior axillary line and heart sounds were soft with no added sounds. Abdominal and neurological examinations were normal.

INVESTIGATIONS
Routine investigation results

Urine	SpG 1.015	Pr neg	Glu neg	Ke neg	Blood neg
Serum	Na 138	K 4.2	HCO_3 26	U 4.5	Cr 97
	Alb 36	Bil 7	AAT 19	AP 94	γGT 16
Blood	Hb 148	MCV 83	WCC 11.2	Plt 340	ESR 6

Additional investigations

Arterial blood gases (breathing air) were as follows:

pH	pO_2	pCO_2	$sHCO_3$
7.50	8.9	3.0	26

His chest radiograph (Fig. 35.1) was diagnostic.

Fig. 35.1
Chest radiograph showing a large right pneumothorax with collapse of the right lung and deviation of the mediastinum to the left indicating tension.

DIAGNOSIS

The history of sudden-onset pleuritic chest pain followed by increasing breathlessness with an associated reduction in the intensity of pain is typical of pneumothorax. Mr Currie was extremely distressed and the clinical signs of deviation of the trachea and mediastinum suggest that he had developed a tension pneumothorax. This was confirmed by the radiograph showing a hyperlucent right lung field with displacement of the mediastinum to the left. Tension pneumothorax is an acute medical emergency requiring urgent treatment to prevent cardiorespiratory failure.

OUTCOME

As an emergency measure, a large-bore intravenous cannula was inserted into the right chest anteriorly, allowing decompression of the tension pneumothorax. His extreme distress was relieved almost immediately, and an underwater seal chest drain was subsequently inserted (Fig. 35.2). After 48h, a repeat radiograph showed that his lung remained fully re-expanded. The water seal drain was no longer bubbling or swinging and was therefore removed. A further radiograph was performed 24h later to confirm that the lung remained expanded and he was allowed home.

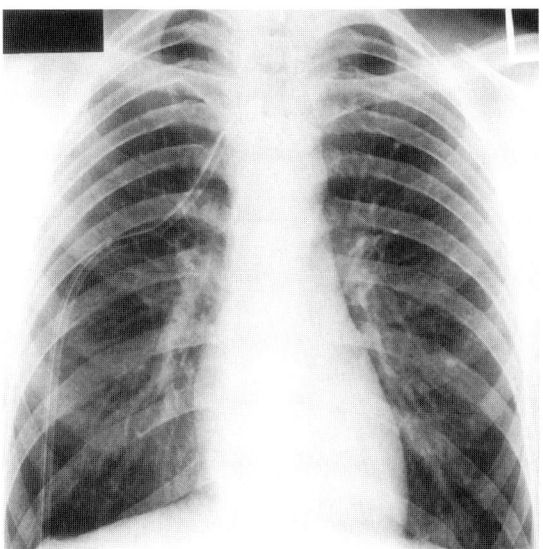

Fig. 35.2
Chest radiograph after insertion of a chest drainage tube in the right pleural space. The right lung has re-expanded.

KEY POINTS

History/Examination
- Sudden onset of pleuritic pain in a previously fit individual may be due to pneumothorax.
- Reduction in severity of the pain as breathlessness increases is typical of pneumothorax.

Investigations
- Most pneumothoraces can be visualized on a standard chest radiograph.

Outcome
- A small pneumothorax may resolve without treatment.
- Treatment is required if the pneumothorax is large enough to cause breathlessness.
- Tension pneumothorax is an acute medical emergency requiring urgent decompression.

Margaret Johnson (78)
Jaundice/abdominal pain

CASE HISTORY
Mrs Johnson, a widow, was admitted to hospital after feeling unwell for 2 days, during which she had had several episodes of abdominal pain under the right ribs. The pain varied in severity and was associated with recurrent shivering and sweating attacks. Her appetite had been poor and she had been nauseated with occasional vomiting. She mentioned that during these 2 days, her urine had appeared very dark in colour.

She had previously been in quite good health, although she was overweight. She lived independently in sheltered housing with assistance from her two daughters who lived nearby.

EXAMINATION
She looked unwell, icteric and dehydrated, and was febrile (37.8°C). There were no cutaneous stigmata of chronic liver disease nor any evidence of scratch marks. Her pulse was 118/min and regular, and blood pressure was 134/80. Her chest was clinically normal. Abdominal examination revealed some tenderness in the right upper quadrant which was exacerbated on inspiration. There was no guarding. The liver, spleen and kidneys were not palpable and there were no other abdominal masses. Bowel sounds and neurological examination were normal.

INVESTIGATIONS
Routine investigation results

Urine	SpG 1.004	Pr neg	Glu neg	Ke ++	Blood neg
Serum	Na 130	K 3.9	HCO$_3$ 22	U 9.8	Cr 138
	Alb 34	Bil 112	AAT 47	AP 756	γGT 489
Blood	Hb 113	MCV 90	WCC 18.9	Plt 300	ESR 78

Additional investigations
Urinary bilirubin was positive (+++) and urobilinogen negative. The prothrombin time was 19 s (reference range 12–16) and serum amylase 256 U/l (reference range < 340). Blood cultures isolated Gram-negative bacilli, later confirmed as *Escherichia coli*. Culture of a mid-stream sample of urine was negative. The plain abdominal and chest radiographs were normal. An abdominal ultrasound scan was abnormal (Fig. 36.1), and endoscopic retrograde cholangiopancreatography (ERCP) confirmed the presence of a stone in the common bile duct (Fig. 36.2).

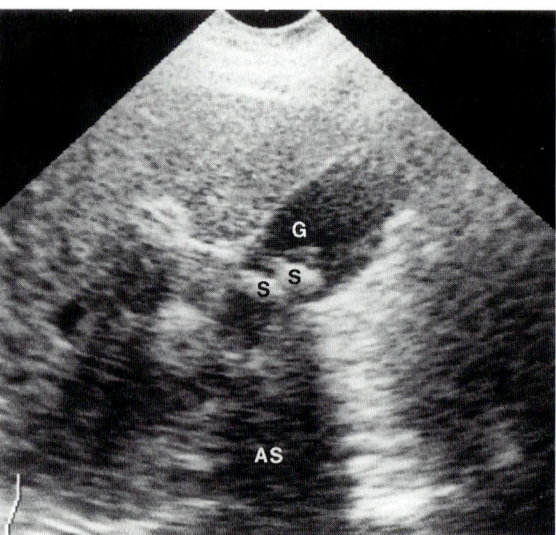

Fig. 36.1
Right parasagittal ultrasound scan section of the upper abdomen showing the gallbladder (G) containing gallstones (S) casting acoustic shadows (AS).

DIAGNOSIS
The history of recurrent sweating and shivering attacks (rigors) is suggestive of bacteraemia. The presence of jaundice and right upper quadrant pain and tenderness suggest that the diagnosis is acute cholangitis. Impaction of a stone in the common bile duct has resulted in biliary tree obstruction leading to biliary colic and obstructive jaundice. The presence of bilirubin in the urine and the disproportionate elevation of serum alkaline phosphatase and γ-glutamyl transferase in relation to the transaminases is in keeping with obstructive jaundice. Dilatation of the

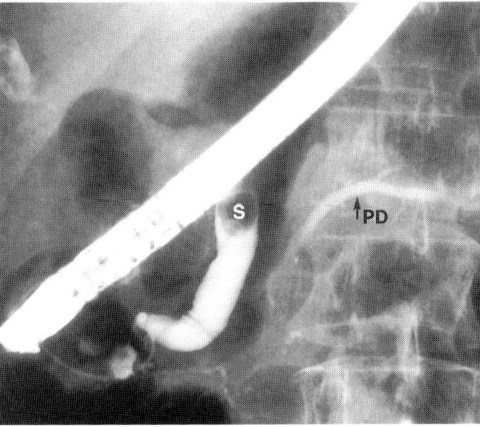

Fig. 36.2
ERCP showing a gallstone (S) in the common bile duct and a normal pancreatic duct (PD).

biliary system and biliary stasis predisposes to biliary infection.

The other common cause of obstructive jaundice in this age group is carcinoma of the head of pancreas, but this is usually painless. The normal serum amylase effectively excludes associated pancreatitis.

An ultrasound scan is a useful investigation to distinguish intrahepatic cholestasis from the extrahepatic cholestasis present in this case. ERCP is used to delineate the site of obstruction in the biliary tree and, when combined with sphincterotomy, may avoid the need for laparotomy in an unwell, elderly patient.

OUTCOME
Mrs Johnson was treated with intravenous antibiotics, fluids and analgesics. Her fever resolved but her jaundice persisted until she underwent endoscopic sphincterotomy and extraction of the stone in the common bile duct.

KEY POINTS

History/Examination
- Jaundice accompanied by rigors suggests biliary tract infection.

Investigations
- The presence of large amounts of bilirubin in the urine and absence of urobilinogen is typical of obstructive jaundice.
- High serum alkaline phosphatase and γ-glutamyl transpeptidase with more modestly elevated transaminases suggests obstructive jaundice.
- Ultrasound scanning is the primary means of evaluating the presence of stones in the gallbladder and biliary tree.

Outcome
- Diagnostic and therapeutic procedures may be combined when sphincterotomy is performed with ERCP.

George Collins (61)
Thirst/polyuria

CASE HISTORY
Mr Collins presented to his general practitioner with increasing thirst over the previous 2 weeks. He had also been getting up at least twice during the night to pass urine. His sister and his late mother suffered from diabetes and he feared that he may now be developing the same trouble. On questioning he admitted to recent tiredness and had possibly lost a few pounds in weight. His appetite had been poor and he had been unusually constipated; he had no dyspeptic symptoms despite having had surgery for a perforated peptic ulcer in his twenties. He denied any chest pain, cough, haemoptysis or breathlessness but admitted to having been less able to keep up with his workmates at the carpet factory where he was a labourer.

He smoked 20 cigarettes per day, drank whisky at weekends (approximately 12 units/week) and was not on regular medication. He was sent to hospital for further assessment after his general practitioner tested his urine.

EXAMINATION
He was lean and looked unwell. His fingers were tar-stained and he had finger clubbing (Fig. 37.1). His tongue was coated and his mouth dry. There was no lymphadenopathy. His pulse was 76/min and regular, blood pressure was 134/74 and the heart sounds were normal. His chest was hyperinflated with prolonged vesicular expiratory sounds but no added sounds. His abdomen was soft and non-tender with no palpable masses; a smooth liver edge was felt 2 cm below the costal margin. There were no neurological abnormalities.

INVESTIGATIONS
Routine investigation results

Urine	SpG 1.018	Pr tr	Glu neg	Ke neg	Blood neg
Serum	Na 139	K 4.7	HCO3 27	U 12.1	Cr 140
	Alb 34	Bil 14	AAT 27	AP 103	γGT 34
Blood	Hb 138	MCV 91	WCC 7.7	Plt 312	ESR 39

Additional investigations
The chest radiograph was abnormal (Fig. 37.2). Random plasma glucose was 7.2 mmol/l (reference range < 8.0) and serum calcium was 3.12 mmol/l

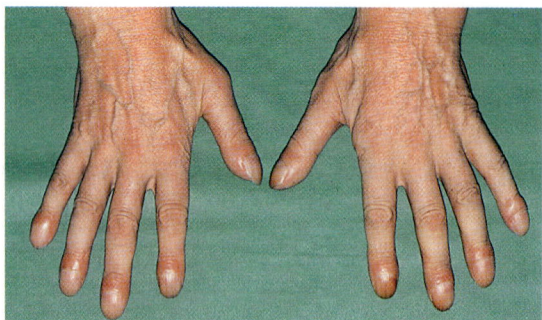

Fig. 37.1
Photograph of hands showing finger clubbing and tar staining.

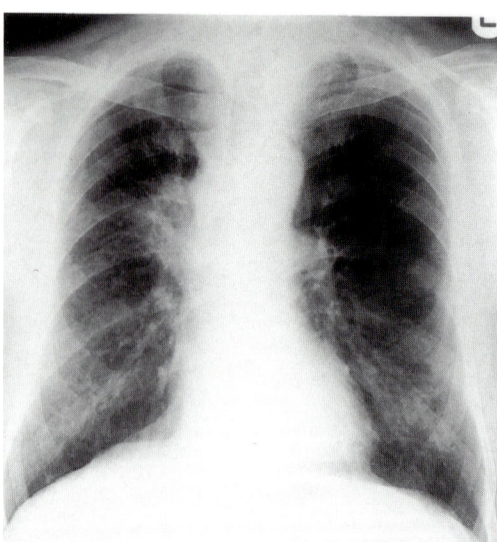

Fig. 37.2
Chest radiograph showing a mass at the upper pole of the right hilum.

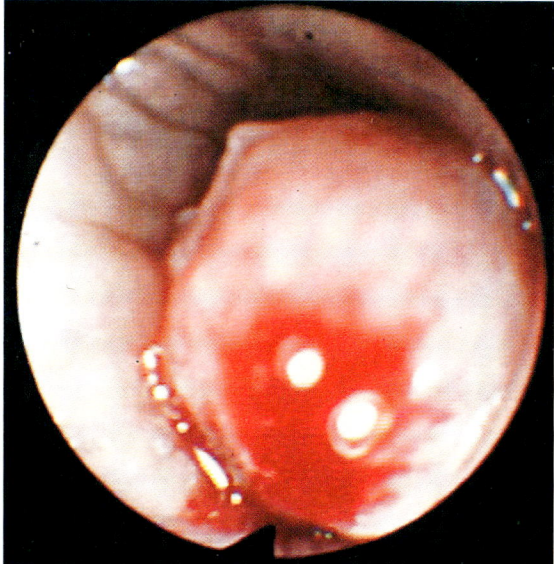

Fig. 37.3
Bronchoscopic view showing tumour mass with bleeding at site of biopsy.

(2.20–2.60). Sputum cytology showed no abnormal cells. Bronchoscopic appearances are shown in Fig. 37.3; histology of the bronchoscopic biopsy showed squamous carcinoma.

DIAGNOSIS

Thirst and polyuria, while most commonly due to diabetes mellitus, can have a number of other causes including chronic renal failure, diabetes insipidus, hypokalaemia, hypercalcaemia and hysterical polydipsia. In this case it was due to hypercalcaemia, which can also produce anorexia and constipation. The patient's tiredness and weight loss, smoking history and finger clubbing were the important clues to its underlying cause. The mass seen on the chest radiograph was characteristic of bronchial carcinoma, and the patient had humoral hypercalcaemia of malignancy owing to production by the tumour of an abnormal substance with parathyroid hormone-like activity. The primary diagnosis was confirmed by bronchoscopic appearances and histological examination of a bronchial biopsy; this showed squamous carcinoma, which is the type of bronchial tumour most commonly associated with hypercalcaemia. Sputum cytology, while very helpful when positive, did not provide any useful information in this case.

His liver was palpable as a result of downward displacement by his hyperinflated lungs rather than of metastatic disease, and the abnormal renal function tests were due to dehydration caused by the hypercalcaemic diuresis.

OUTCOME

The hypercalcaemia was corrected by intravenous fluids, loop diuretic and bisphosphonate injection, with relief of symptoms and recovery of renal function. In the absence of demonstrable metastatic disease he proceeded to pneumonectomy. He returned to work within 3 months and remained well 2 years later. He had stopped smoking.

KEY POINTS

History/Examination
- Thirst and polyuria are symptoms of hypercalcaemia.
- Bronchial carcinoma should always be considered in unwell, middle-aged smokers.

Investigations
- The absence of glycosuria excludes hyperglycaemia as a cause of thirst and polyuria.
- Measure serum calcium (and potassium) levels when the diagnosis of thirst and polyuria is not due to glycosuria.
- Chest radiography is an important screening investigation in the assessment of ill patients.

Outcome
- The presence of a metabolic manifestation of malignant disease does not necessarily preclude successful treatment of the primary condition.

Alexander Gunn (48)
Abdominal pain

CASE HISTORY

Mr Gunn was celebrating his daughter's engagement, and consumed about eight pints of beer and six double whiskies during the course of the evening. The following day he awoke with a 'hangover' and an aching pain in the epigastric region. He took some antacid mixture and a glass of milk and left for work. Later in the day his pain was increasing so he returned home to rest. After arriving home he vomited on several occasions, producing a mixture of watery fluid and altered food but no blood. He took some antacid without relief and during the following night he became agitated with increasingly severe pain. When his wife noticed that he had become confused, she realised that this was more serious than a hangover. She called his general practitioner and he was admitted to hospital.

He had a history of a duodenal ulcer treated with an H_2–receptor blocker 5 years previously. During the past year, he had suffered intermittent episodes of dull epigastric pain which were partially relieved by antacids. He was employed as a driver for a brewing company, making deliveries to hotels and public houses. He smoked 50 cigarettes daily and admitted to drinking three pints of beer and two whiskies every night. He had a family history of peptic ulcer, his father and one uncle having been affected. He was married with three children.

EXAMINATION

He was confused, agitated and distressed with abdominal pain. There was tar staining of his fingers but no clubbing. He appeared dehydrated with loss of skin turgor, and was pyrexial (38.8°C). His peripheries were cold with poor capillary return. His pulse was 120/min, regular and of small volume, and blood pressure was 90/70. His heart sounds were soft with no added sounds or murmurs, and peripheral pulses were absent distal to the femorals bilaterally. In his chest, there was dullness to percussion at the left base and diminished breath sounds and vocal resonance over the same region. His abdomen was distended and there was discoloration in both flanks (Fig. 38.1). The abdomen was rigid and tender on direct palpation with associated rebound tenderness. There were no palpable abdominal masses and bowel sounds were absent. Rectal examination was normal and the faecal occult blood test was negative. He was disorientated in time and place, but there were no focal neurological abnormalities.

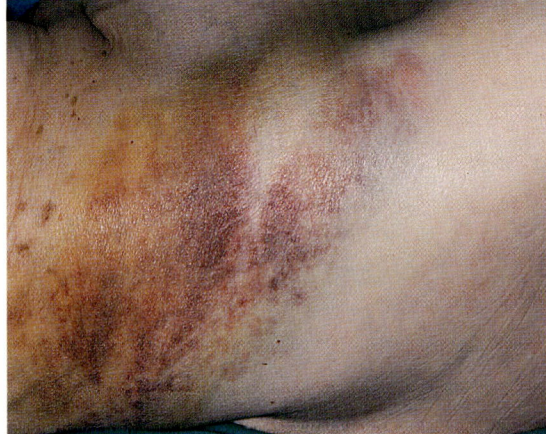

Fig. 38.1
Grey-Turner's sign.

INVESTIGATIONS
Routine investigation results

Urine	SpG 1015	Pr neg	Glu +	Ke neg	Blood neg
Serum	Na 135	K 3.2	HCO_3 20	U 18	Cr 170
	Alb 31	Bil 36	AAT 67	AP 105	γGT 74
Blood	Hb 155	MCV 98	WCC 18.6	Plt 540	ESR 47

Additional investigations

Serum amylase was 1503 U/l (reference range < 340), serum calcium 1.81 mmol/l (2.2–2.6) and blood glucose 10 mmol/l (< 8). Blood cultures were sterile. Arterial blood gases (breathing air) were as follows:

pH	pO$_2$	pCO$_2$	sHCO$_3$
7.34	6.8	3.1	20

A chest radiograph showed evidence of a small left pleural effusion. Ultrasound scanning of the abdomen revealed no evidence of gallstones, but the liver echo pattern was suggestive of fatty infiltration. The pancreas was largely obscured owing to bowel gas, but was visualized on CT scanning (Fig. 38.2).

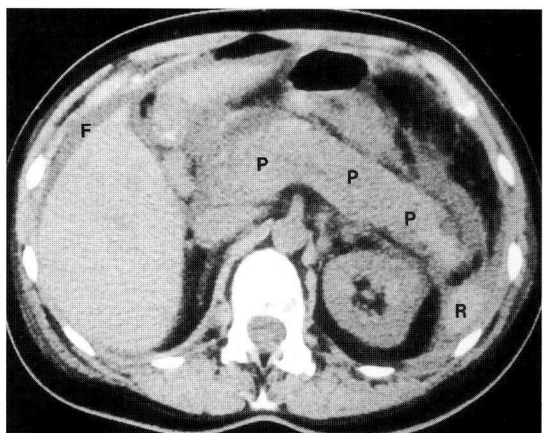

Fig. 38.2
Single transverse CT scan through the abdomen at the level of the pancreas, showing an enlarged pancreas (P) free peritoneal fluid (F) and retroperitoneal fluid (R).

DIAGNOSIS

The patient had a rigid tender abdomen with absent bowel sounds, the signs of an 'acute abdomen'. Bruising in the flanks (Grey-Turner's sign) suggests the diagnosis of acute pancreatitis and this is confirmed by the very high serum amylase. Acute pancreatitis often follows a large intake of alcohol and is a serious, potentially fatal condition. The findings of cold peripheries, tachycardia and hypotension indicated that he was shocked, and the confusion and clouding of consciousness were a consequence of poor cerebral blood flow and hypoxia.

The arterial blood gas results confirmed that he was hypoxic, and also show evidence of a metabolic acidosis, which was a result of poor tissue perfusion. The elevated blood urea and creatinine signify renal failure, which may occur in up to one-fifth of patients with pancreatitis. Fever and the elevated white cell count and ESR are related to pancreatic necrosis and do not necessarily imply infection, although secondary infection with bacteraemia or cholangitis may occur. Elevation of blood glucose and glycosuria commonly occur in pancreatitis. The reduction in serum calcium (a true reduction, even when corrected for the low albumin) is associated with a poor prognosis. The abnormalities of liver function may be in part due to the acute pancreatitis and in part to his history of excessive alcohol consumption with associated alcoholic liver damage.

Abdominal ultrasound is the imaging technique of first choice, but in this case the pancreas could not be visualized adequately owing to excessive bowel gas. CT scanning, however, showed pancreatic swelling.

In this case, the precipitating cause is alcohol ingestion, although there are a number of other causes of pancreatitis including biliary tract disease, infectious disease (e.g. mumps), drugs (azathioprine and corticosteroids) and surgery or instrumentation of the biliary tract as in ERCP.

OUTCOME

He was treated with oxygen and intravenous fluids and a nasogastric tube was inserted. Broad-spectrum intravenous antibiotics were given. His haemodynamic state, blood gases and urine output were closely monitored. Despite intensive supportive therapy, he developed progressive respiratory and renal failure with disseminated intravascular coagulation, and he died 7 days after admission.

KEY POINTS

History/Examination
- Excessive alcohol intake may cause acute pancreatitis.
- Bruising in the flanks or around the umbilicus suggests haemorrhagic pancreatitis.

Investigations
- Marked elevation of the serum amylase is highly suggestive of pancreatitis.
- Hypocalcaemia, renal failure and respiratory failure are associated with a poor prognosis.

Outcome
- Acute pancreatitis has a significant mortality.

39 James Murray (44) Chest pain

CASE HISTORY

Mr Murray, a cattleman, was admitted to hospital with a 24 h history of dry cough and sharp left-sided chest pain. The pain was severe and was worsened by breathing or coughing. He had tried paracetamol, but this had virtually no effect on the pain. In addition to the pain, he felt generally unwell, breathless and feverish and had a dull headache. His general practitioner saw him at home and decided to admit him to hospital immediately.

Mr Murray had been in good health, although 14 years ago he had had brucellosis diagnosed by the local infectious disease physicians. He was married with two children and lived near the cattle farm. None of his family or the farm staff had recently been ill. He had not recently been abroad. He smoked 40 cigarettes per day and took alcohol only occasionally. He was not taking medication.

EXAMINATION

He was febrile (39.9°C), confused and sweating profusely. Lesions were noted on his lips (Fig. 39.1). His fauces were normal, and he had no cervical lymphadenopathy. His pulse was 120/min and regular, and blood pressure was 130/60. Respiratory system examination revealed central cyanosis and tachypnoea. There was dullness to percussion at the left base extending into the axilla, and auscultation over this area revealed bronchial breathing, increased vocal resonance and a harsh pleural friction rub. The remainder of the examination was normal.

INVESTIGATIONS
Routine investigation results

Urine	SpG 1.010	Pr +	Glu neg	Ke +	Blood neg
Serum	Na 135	K 4.9	HCO₃ 20	U 6.0	Cr 101
	Alb 33	Bil 24	AAT 45	AP 79	γGT 56
Blood	Hb 135	MCV 91	WCC 24.5	Plt 550	ESR 51

Additional investigations

Arterial blood gases (breathing air) were as follows:

pH	pO_2	pCO_2	$sHCO_3$
7.46	6.5	3.0	25

The chest radiograph was abnormal (Fig. 39.2). A blood film showed a neutrophil leucocytosis. Sputum microscopy and Gram stain showed numerous pus cells and Gram-positive diplococci, which were later confirmed to be *Streptococcus pneumoniae*. The sputum and serum latex agglutination tests for pneumoccocal

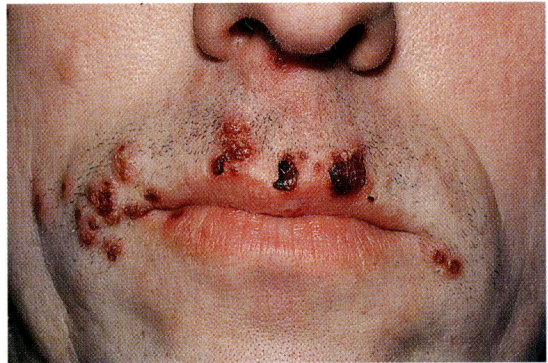

Fig. 39.1
Herpes labialis.

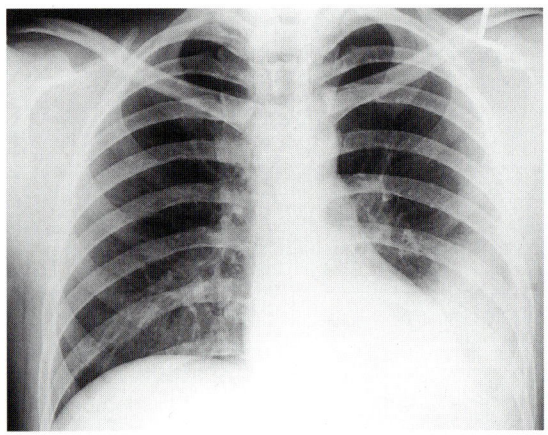

Fig. 39.2
Chest radiograph showing opacification of the left lower lobe. The left hemidiaphragm cannot be identified.

antigen were negative. Blood cultures grew *Strep. pneumoniae.*

DIAGNOSIS

The short history of pleuritic chest pain associated with fever, often with rigors, dyspnoea and non-productive cough, is suggestive of respiratory infection. Dullness to percussion with associated bronchial breathing and increased vocal resonance are signs of consolidation, typical of lobar pneumonia, which in this case was due to *Strep. pneumoniae* (pneumococcal pneumonia). Herpes labialis (Fig 39.1) is a common associated finding with pneumococcal pneumonia. The cough often becomes productive within 48–72 h and a pinkish or rusty coloration of the sputum is common (Fig. 39.3).

The arterial blood gases showed hypoxaemia, indicating respiratory failure, and there were minor abnormalities of liver function which are common in association with severe infection. The diagnosis was confirmed by the positive blood and sputum cultures. Although antigen detection by immunoelectrophoresis or latex agglutination in sputum, blood or urine can be a means of rapid diagnosis, the test lacks sensitivity and was negative in this case.

Strep. pneumoniae is the commonest cause of community-acquired pneumonia in the UK. Other organisms that may cause a lobar pneumonia include *Mycoplasma pneumoniae, Staphylococcus aureus, Legionella pneumophila, Chlamydia pneumoniae* and, less commonly, *Klebsiella pneumoniae* and other Gram-negative bacilli. Lobar pneumonia is a potentially fatal condition, a poor prognosis being more likely in the elderly and in subjects who are confused or have an elevated blood urea at the time of presentation.

OUTCOME

Mr Murray was treated with intravenous benzylpenicillin, 60% oxygen and analgesics. His pleuritic pain resolved and he became afebrile over the following 3 days, during which he developed a productive cough. He made a gradual recovery, although he lost 6 kg in weight during the course of his illness and was unable to return to work for 5 weeks after the onset of symptoms. His chest radiograph 2 months later still showed some residual shadowing at the left base, but 6 months later it had returned to normal.

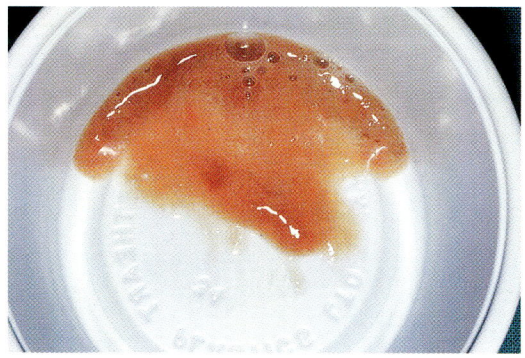

Fig. 39.3
'Rusty' sputum.

KEY POINTS

History/Examination
- The abrupt onset of fever and pleuritic chest pain is typical of lobar pneumonia.
- *Strep. pneumoniae* is the commonest cause of lobar pneumonia in the UK.

Investigations
- Rapid diagnosis may be made by Gram stain of sputum or by detection of pneumococcal antigen.
- Blood cultures are positive in one-third of cases of pneumococcal pneumonia.

Outcome
- Resolution of radiographic changes in lobar pneumonia may take weeks or months.

John Austin (28) Swelling

CASE HISTORY

Mr Austin presented as an emergency via the Casualty Department late one evening complaining of progressive swelling and discomfort of his legs over the previous 2 weeks. He had also noted some facial puffiness and had been unusually tired and breathless on minor exertion. He had noted no change in appetite or bowel habit, no dysuria or frequency, and no cold intolerance.

He denied any previous illness of note apart from 'bad skin' as a child. He did not know anything of his family, having been adopted as a baby. He had lost touch with his adoptive family for several years and had no close friends. Although he had been designated educationally subnormal, he lived independently, working in a kitchen and living in a room in lodgings. He smoked 15 cigarettes per day but did not drink alcohol. He had not been taking any drugs over the previous 24 h, other than aspirin for the discomfort in his legs.

EXAMINATION

Mr Austin had facial swelling and marked pitting oedema of his legs (Fig. 40.1), abdominal wall and hands. He was not distressed at rest and not unduly pale. He was apyrexial but his hands were warm and his skin rather dry, particularly over the elbows. There was no lymphadenopathy and no goitre. The jugular venous pressure was not elevated. His pulse was 88/min and regular, and blood pressure was 112/72 supine, falling to 96/60 on standing. The heart sounds were normal. There was some dullness to percussion at the lung bases. The abdomen was rather tense and shifting dullness was detectable. There was no hepatosplenomegaly and no tenderness in the renal angles. There were no neurological abnormalities and fundoscopy was normal.

INVESTIGATIONS
Routine investigation results

Urine	SpG 1.032	Pr ++++	Glu neg	Ke neg	Blood neg
Serum	Na 133	K 4.2	HCO3 26	U 3.6	Cr 79
	Alb 12	Bil 4	AAT 36	AP 87	γGT 22
Blood	Hb 145	MCV 88	WCC 5.6	Plt 437	ESR 18

Additional investigations

A mid-stream specimen of urine contained no pus cells or casts and produced no growth on culture. A 24 h urine collection contained 11.4 g of protein (reference range < 0.15) and had a sodium content of 12 mmol (100–250). Total serum cholesterol was 12.3 mmol/l (4.0–7.2), total serum thyroxine 41 nmol/l (70–150), TSH 2.2 mU/l (0.35–3.3), and serum C3 complement level 50 mg/l (25–70).

A chest radiograph showed pleural fluid at both lung bases, and an abdominal ultrasound scan showed free intra-abdominal fluid but normal liver, spleen and kidneys.

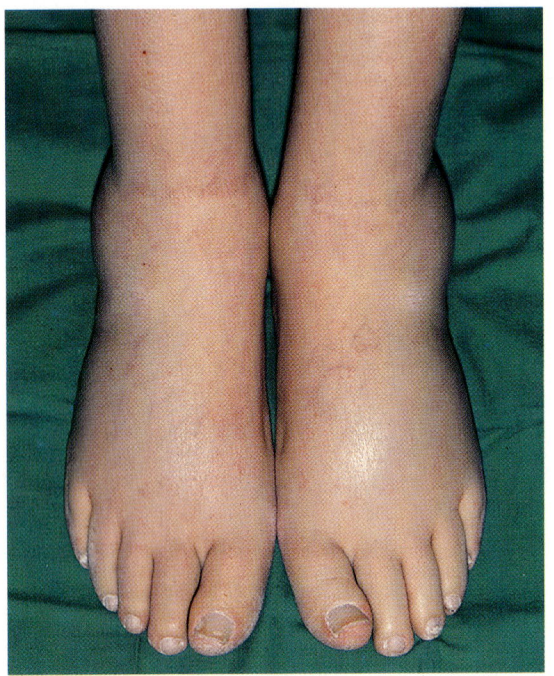

Fig. 40.1
Marked oedema of feet and ankles.

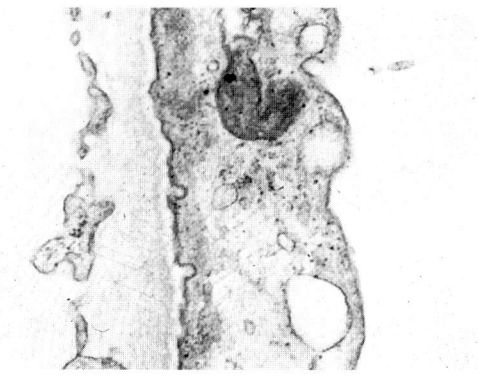
(a)

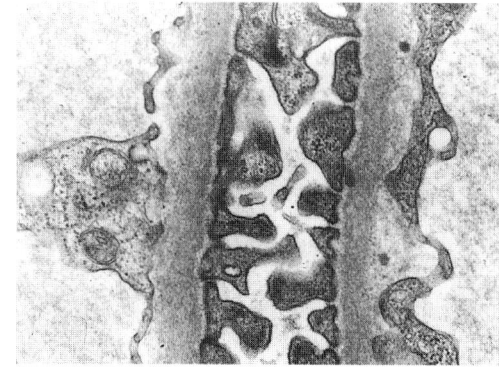
(b)

Fig. 40.2
(a) Electron micrograph of glomerular tissue showing the podocyte fusion that is characteristic of minimal-change nephropathy.
(b) Normal electron micrograph for comparison showing well preserved podocyte structure.

DIAGNOSIS

Oedema in dependent sites is a feature of severe acquired hypoalbuminaemia, which can occur as a result of malnutrition, malabsorption, reduced hepatic albumin synthesis, or excessive protein loss from the gut or in the urine. This patient had gross proteinuria as part of the nephrotic syndrome and presented with a widespread increase in extracellular fluid including pleural effusions and ascites. A renal biopsy under ultrasound control showed histologically normal tissue on light microscopy, but the podocyte fusion on electron microscopy (Fig. 40.2) confirmed a diagnosis of so-called minimal-change nephropathy. This condition, which accounts for most cases of childhood nephrotic syndrome and around a quarter of cases in adults, has a comparatively good prognosis with the great majority responding favourably to glucocorticoid therapy. The absence of urinary casts or lowered C3 complement levels were inconsistent with a diagnosis of glomerulonephritis and there was no history of ingestion of any drug known to cause nephrotic syndrome.

The significant postural drop in blood pressure indicated intravascular volume depletion; the low urinary sodium reflected renal salt conservation in an attempt to maintain intravascular volume. A high serum cholesterol is a recognized feature of nephrotic syndrome, which resolves with effective treatment of the renal lesion. The low total serum thyroxine level was an indication of reduced levels of thyroxine-binding proteins; the normal TSH level excluded primary hypothyroidism.

OUTCOME

Mr Austin was treated with oral loop and potassium-sparing diuretics and, on confirmation of the diagnosis, with oral prednisolone. He was also treated with subcutaneous heparin in view of the high risk of venous thrombosis. His oedema improved over the following 2 weeks as his serum albumin rose to 20 g/l. Four weeks after discharge from hospital he was re-admitted with a clinical relapse and an albumin of 11 g/l. He admitted to poor compliance with medication.

KEY POINTS

History/Examination
- Consider hypoalbuminaemia as a cause of dependent oedema.
- Ascites and pleural effusions occur in hypoalbuminaemic patients owing to the accumulation of extracellular fluid in the body cavities.

Investigations
- The diagnosis of nephrotic syndrome was confirmed by urinary protein measurement.
- Renal biopsy with electron microscopy is necessary to reach a diagnosis of minimal-change nephropathy.

Outcome
- Minimal-change nephropathy generally responds well to steroid therapy.
- Failure of patients to comply with prescribed medication is a major problem in clinical practice.

Agnes Campbell (69) Collapse

CASE HISTORY

Mrs Campbell was a rather eccentric lady who lived alone in a small cottage in the countryside, keeping hens, a cow and a variety of dogs and cats. She made a weekly trip to the local town to buy provisions, and her only other contact with the outside world was via the postman. During one particularly severe spell of winter weather, the postman called on Mrs Campbell and received no reply. He called the local police and a search was instituted. Mrs Campbell was found about 200 m from the house, lying in a hedgerow in a semi-conscious state, and was transferred immediately to hospital. She was unable to give any coherent history.

Her case records revealed that she had undergone hysterectomy for uterine fibroids 20 years previously, and that she had been prescribed a major tranquillizer for 30 years for a diagnosis of paranoid schizophrenia. She was known to drink about one bottle of sherry per month, and was a non-smoker.

EXAMINATION

She was drowsy and uncooperative, and appeared cold and peripherally cyanosed. Her temperature, measured by rectal thermometer, was 29°C. Her pulse was 40/min, regular and of small volume, and blood pressure was 100/60. The heart sounds were present but soft. Her peripheries were extremely cold, with impalpable pulses. Her feet showed gross signs of neglect with marked deformities of the toenails (onychogryphosis) (Fig. 41.1). Her respiratory rate was 7/min and there were some coarse crackles at the right lung base. Her abdomen was soft and non-tender and bowel sounds were very infrequent. She had few detectable focal neurological signs, although cooperation with examination was limited. Sensation was difficult to test, but she did not withdraw her feet in response to pin prick suggesting that sensation was diminished. Tendon reflexes were generally diminished.

INVESTIGATIONS
Routine investigation results

Urine	SpG 1010	Pr tr	Glu neg	Ke +	Blood neg
Serum	Na 130	K 5.2	HCO$_3$ 18	U 15.0	Cr 155
	Alb 36	Bil 17	AAT 30	AP 110	γGT 30
Blood	Hb 130	MCV 88	WCC 13.5	Plt 390	ESR 3

Additional investigations
An ECG showed a number of abnormal features (Fig. 41.2). Blood alcohol was 0.7 g/l and serum amylase was 500 U/l (reference range < 340).

DIAGNOSIS
The primary diagnosis is hypothermia. This may occur in individuals, especially the elderly, exposed to low

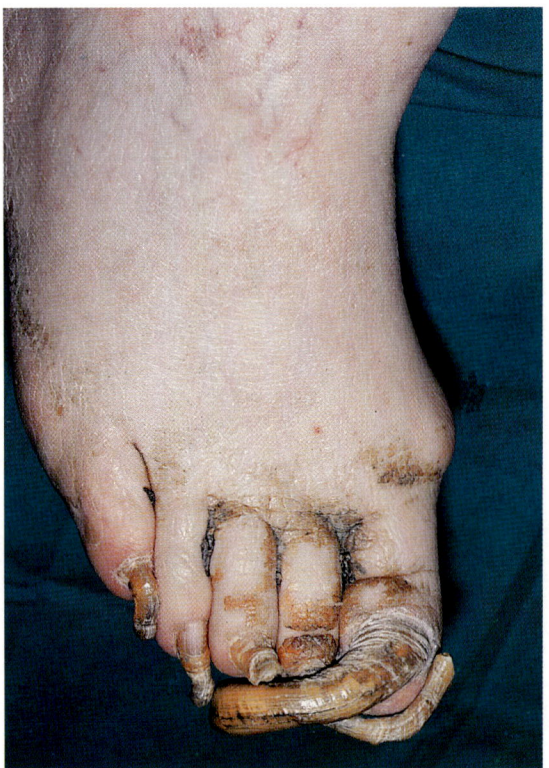

Fig. 41.1
Onychogryphosis.

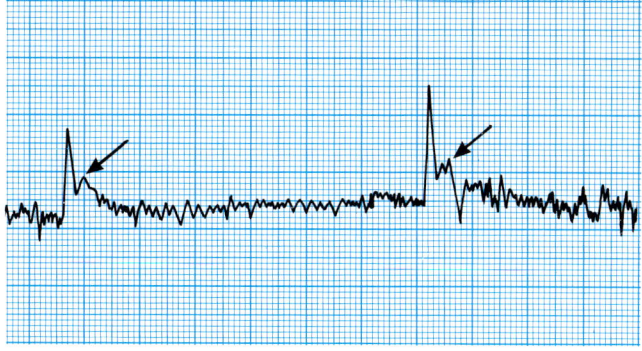

Fig. 41.2
ECG rhythm strip showing bradycardia, shivering artefact and J waves (arrowed).

temperatures for prolonged periods. In Mrs Campbell's case, however, there are two additional contributing causes, namely the use of major tranquillizers and ingestion of alcohol, both of which cause peripheral vasodilatation and speed the rate of heat loss from the body.

Bradycardia and slow respiration are characteristic of hypothermia, and cardiorespiratory arrest is particularly likely when the core temperature is below 29°C. The serum amylase is frequently elevated and frank pancreatitis may occur. The ECG changes are typical, with a sinus bradycardia, prolongation of the P–R interval and the presence of 'J waves' (Fig. 41.2). The latter are diagnostic of hypothermia when present, but occur in less than half of all hypothermic patients.

OUTCOME

Attempts were made to prevent further heat loss and to promote rewarming by wrapping the patient in a thermal blanket. Heart rate and rectal temperature were monitored and intravenous fluids warmed to body temperature were given. Blood glucose and serum potassium were monitored as both hypoglycaemia and hyperkalaemia may occur during recovery.

Two hours after admission, Mrs Campbell developed ventricular fibrillation (Fig. 41.3) from which she could not be resuscitated.

KEY POINTS

History/Examination
- The elderly are at risk of hypothermia.
- Hypothermia may be exacerbated by drugs and alcohol.
- Core temperature should be measured using a low reading thermometer.

Investigations
- Acidosis, hypoglycaemia, hyperkalaemia and elevation of serum amylase may all occur in hypothermia.
- ECG monitoring is important in view of the risk of cardiac arrhythmias.

Outcome
- Hypothermia carries a high mortality in the elderly.

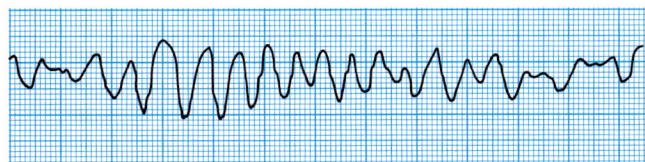

Fig. 41.3
ECG rhythm strip showing ventricular fibrillation.

David Smith (68)
Shingles

CASE HISTORY

Mr Smith developed severe pain in the right lower chest which was continuous and not relieved by paracetamol. He had no cough or sputum and was puzzled as to the cause of the pain since he had been previously well and did not recollect injuring his chest. About 2 days after the onset of the pain, he developed a red rash over the right lower chest and decided to contact his general practitioner. He denied any other recent symptoms but mentioned that he had noticed a small, painless swelling in the left armpit while having a bath some 4 months previously. Although this had gradually enlarged, it was not causing any discomfort and he had therefore not brought it to the attention of his general practitioner.

Mr Smith took no medication and did not smoke. He was a retired factory worker and lived with his wife. He admitted drinking up to six pints of beer each week.

EXAMINATION

He was lean, afebrile and in some discomfort from the vesicular erythematous rash over the T6 dermatome on the right (Fig. 42.1). There was generalized painless bilateral inguinal and axillary lymphadenopathy (Fig. 42.2). His pulse was 75/min and regular, and blood pressure was 150/90. His heart sounds were normal and there were no murmurs. Respiratory examination was limited by chest pain but was otherwise normal. Abdominal examination revealed a smooth, non-tender spleen palpable 2 cm below the costal margin. The remainder of the examination was normal.

INVESTIGATIONS
Routine investigation results

Urine	SpG 1.002	Pr neg	Glu neg	Ke +	Blood neg
Serum	Na 131	K 4.0	HCO₃ 20	U 9.7	Cr 124
	Alb 46	Bil 23	AAT 31	AP 167	γGT 70
Blood	Hb 107	MCV 93	WCC 180	Plt 284	ESR 78

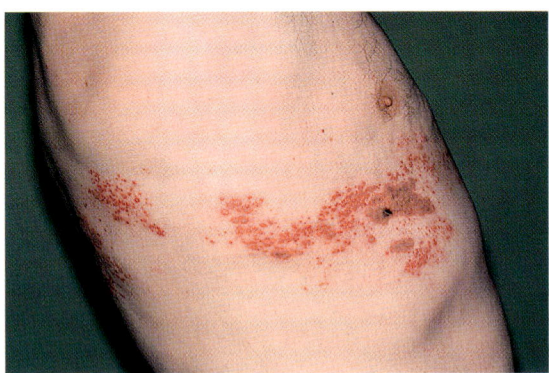

Fig. 42.1
Herpes zoster rash in T6 dermatome.

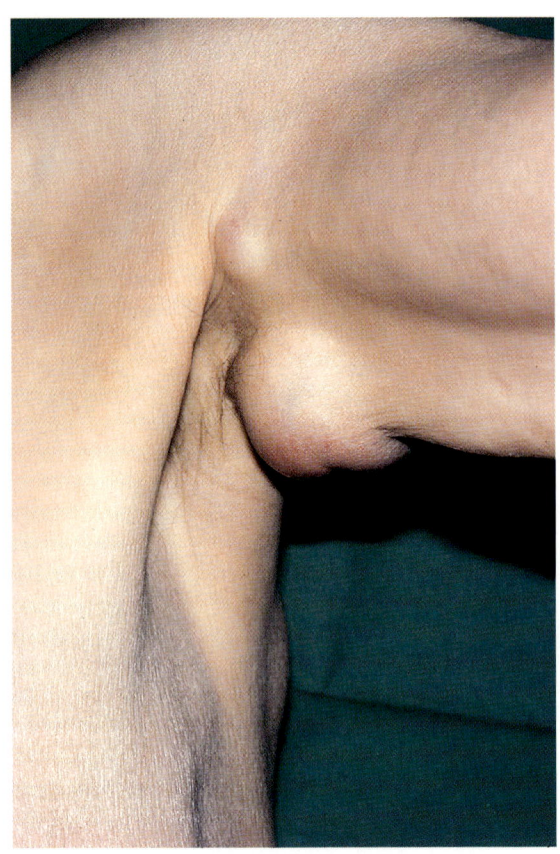

Fig. 42.2
Axillary lymphadenopathy.

Additional investigations

A differential white cell count showed marked lymphocytosis and the blood film suggested the diagnosis (Fig. 42.3). Immunophenotyping confirmed that these lymphocytes were B-cells. Bone marrow trephine and aspiration revealed heavy lymphocytic infiltration of the myeloid tissue. Serum immunoglobulins were: IgG 5.2 g/l (reference range 8–14), IgM 0.3 g/l (0.5–2.5), IgA 0.7 g/l (0.9–3.5). The chest radiograph was normal.

DIAGNOSIS

Severe pain followed by the development of a vesicular rash in a dermatomal distribution is characteristic of shingles (herpes zoster). The rash progresses through a series of stages from macules to vesicles to pustules and eventually forms scabs before resolving. Herpes zoster is often an isolated condition, especially in the elderly, but it may occur in subjects with underlying disease. In this case, the presence of lymphadenopathy together with the very high white cell count suggests the underlying diagnosis of chronic lymphocytic leukaemia (CLL), and this is confirmed by the blood film appearances and the results of immunophenotyping. A moderately enlarged spleen is often found in the early stages of CLL.

Patients with CLL may remain asymptomatic for months or years and may present with constitutional symptoms (50%) such as weight loss, malaise, fever or sweating. In Mr Smith's case, hypogammaglobulinaemia, as evidenced by the low levels of all immunoglobulins, placed him at risk of opportunistic infection.

OUTCOME

Mr Smith was initially treated with analgesics and high-dose oral acyclovir. Once the herpes zoster had resolved, he was treated with chemotherapy and immunoglobulin replacement therapy. During the next few months, he had intermittent episodes of sharp pain in the distribution of the rash (post-herpetic neuralgia).

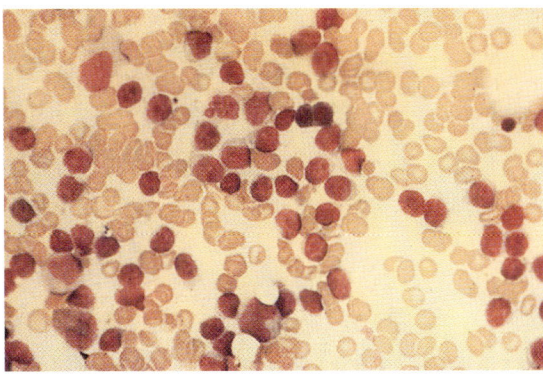

Fig. 42.3
Blood film showing mature abnormal small lymphocytes consistent with CLL.

KEY POINTS

History/Examination
- Pain followed by a vesicular rash in a dermatomal distribution is typical of herpes zoster.
- Herpes zoster may be associated with underlying disease.

Investigations
- The very high white cell count, which is predominantly lymphocytic, is diagnostic of CLL.
- Hypogammaglobulinaemia is a common feature of CLL.

Outcome
- Patients with CLL have a relatively favourable prognosis (median survival 5 years).

Calum Adams (66)
Headaches, collapse

CASE HISTORY

Mr Adams, a barman, was brought to the Emergency Department by one of his customers after he had collapsed at work. The customer said that Mr Adams had been pouring a beer when he suddenly went rigid and fell down behind the bar. He was unable to speak and had 'jerking' movements of his arms and legs. By the time he arrived at the Emergency Department he was drowsy and moaning, but was still unable to give a coherent history. He was admitted to the medical ward for observation and further investigation.

When his son arrived at the hospital, he said that Mr Adams had a long-standing alcohol problem for which he had seen a number of self-help groups and psychiatrists. However, so far as he was aware, Mr Adams had not consumed any alcohol for 2 months. He had recently mentioned that he had been having headaches for the past 3 weeks, worse in the morning and sometimes with associated vomiting. There was no history of head injury but he had had two 'blackouts' in the past fortnight. He had refused to seek help after these episodes.

Mr Adams was divorced with three adult children. He had been in his present employment for 3 years after losing ownership of his own public house due to his alcoholism. He smoked 20 cigarettes daily and previously consumed up to 20 pints of beer per week. He was not taking medication.

EXAMINATION

When initially seen he was drowsy, moaning and holding his head. There was no fever or evidence of head injury. His pulse was 60/min and regular, and blood pressure was 190/90. There were no cardiac murmurs or carotid bruits. Respiratory examination was normal. Neurological examination revealed some drift of the left hand when both arms were extended. There also appeared to be mild weakness of the left leg and the left plantar response was extensor. Sensation was normal although cooperation was limited. The optic fundi were normal.

INVESTIGATIONS
Routine investigation results

Urine	SpG 1.020	Pr neg	Glu neg	Ke neg	Blood neg
Serum	Na 135	K 4.3	HCO_3 25	U 2.5	Cr 98
	Alb 34	Bil 9	AAT 27	AP 71	γGT 58
Blood	Hb 159	MCV 99	WCC 10.9	Plt 387	ESR 18

Additional investigations

Blood ethanol was not detected, and a serum toxicology screen for benzodiazepines, salicylates and paracetamol was negative. Random blood sugar was 5 mmol/l (reference range < 8). Chest and skull radiographs were normal. A CT head scan revealed an abnormality (Fig. 43.1).

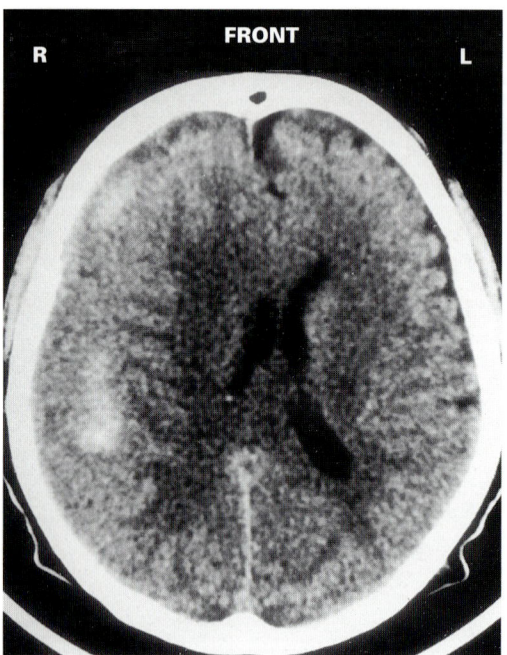

Fig. 43.1
A single transverse CT scan at the level of the lateral ventricles showing a large right subdural haematoma with effacement of the right lateral ventricle. There is midline shift and compression of the underlying cerebral hemisphere.

DIAGNOSIS

The history of headaches that are worse in the morning and associated with vomiting is suggestive of raised intracranial pressure. The description of his collapse suggests a grand mal seizure, which, in a middle-aged man with a background of alcohol excess, is often due to alcohol withdrawal. However, Mr Adams had apparently been abstinent for 2 months and acute alcohol withdrawal is therefore unlikely. The presence of subtle neurological impairment in the left arm and leg and the upgoing plantar response suggest a structural lesion. The diagnosis of subdural haematoma was confirmed by CT scanning. A subdural haematoma can follow even a relatively mild head injury, particularly in alcoholics who are prone to falls during periods of intoxication. In about half the cases of chronic subdural haematoma, no injury is recalled. The most common neurological signs in chronic subdural haematoma are pupillary inequality, long tract signs with motor limb weakness and occasionally an extensor plantar response. In 5–10% of all cases epileptic fits occur.

OUTCOME

He was transferred to the neurosurgical unit where he underwent successful evacuation of the haematoma. He remains well with no long-term neurological sequelae. He has had no further fits but has been hospitalized on two subsequent occasions with acute alcohol intoxication.

KEY POINTS

History/Examination
- An eye-witness account of an episode of collapse is helpful.
- Headache and vomiting are symptoms of a subdural haematoma.
- Neurological abnormalities in subdural haematoma are often subtle.

Investigations
- Remember drugs, alcohol and metabolic disorders may cause altered consciousness and fits.
- CT head scanning is useful to demonstrate space-occupying lesions.

Outcome
- Neurological abnormalities can resolve after evacuation of a subdural haematoma.

44 Thomas Whyte (40) Vomiting blood

CASE HISTORY

Mr Whyte presented at the Emergency Department in the early hours of the morning having vomited blood on several occasions. The previous evening he had attended a golf club dinner and had consumed a lot of alcohol. On his return home he had vomited and then fallen asleep in a chair for an hour or so. He woke feeling nauseated and vomited again, this time bringing up brownish material. As he continued to retch and vomit he started bringing up bright red blood mixed with fluid. He estimated that he had lost one and a half pints of blood. This so alarmed him that he woke his wife and asked her to take him to hospital.

He had never vomited blood before, and had recently kept well with normal appetite and bowel habit, and no change in weight. His two previous hospital admissions were with pneumonia as a teenager, and for observation following a head injury in a road traffic accident a year ago. His younger brother was being treated for Hodgkin's disease and his son had recently recovered from *Salmonella* food poisoning. He worked as a telephone engineer, was a non-smoker, and did not regularly drink alcohol. He was not on regular medication, but occasionally took proprietary antacid tablets.

EXAMINATION

He smelt of alcohol and looked anxious and pale, but had well perfused conjunctivae and mucous membranes. His pulse was 110/min, and blood pressure was 184/102. He was tachypnoeic at around 20 breaths/min but his heart and lungs were normal on auscultation. There was distinct epigastric tenderness, but no palpable abdominal masses or organomegaly. Bowel sounds were normal and faecal occult blood testing was negative.

INVESTIGATIONS
Routine investigation results

Urine	SpG 1.007	Pr neg	Glu neg	Ke tr	Blood neg
Serum	Na 135	K 3.6	HCO$_3$ 28	U 5.3	Cr 78
	Alb 39	Bil 18	AAT 21	AP 88	γGT 33
Blood	Hb 151	MCV 83	WCC 8.1	Plt 322	ESR 13

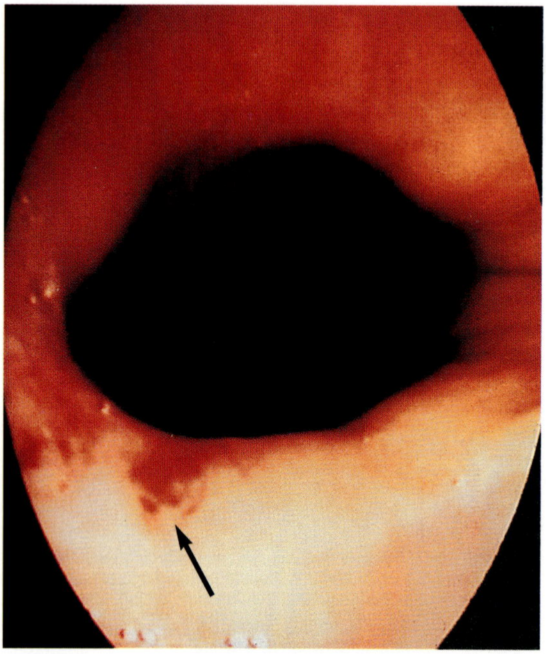

Additional investigations

Blood ethanol level was 1.6 g/l. A chest radiograph was normal, showing no evidence of aspiration of gastric contents or subdiaphragmatic air. The diagnosis was confirmed at endoscopy (Fig. 44.1).

DIAGNOSIS

This man's haematemesis was due to an upper gastrointestinal mucosal tear, which had been caused by the mechanical effects of repeated retching. The diagnosis was strongly suspected on the basis of the history: blood appeared in the vomitus *after* the initial episode of what became protracted retching. The

Fig. 44.1
Endoscopic view of lower oesophagus showing a mucosal tear at the oesophagogastric junction (arrow).

nausea and vomiting were almost certainly as a result of unaccustomed alcohol excess. There were no antecedent symptoms suggesting peptic ulcer, and no history of salicylate or NSAID ingestion to cause acute erosive gastritis, but as neither of these diagnoses can be definitely excluded on history, endoscopy was the only means of establishing the diagnosis. The abdominal tenderness was simply related to the muscular strain of repeated retching.

The patient's skin pallor, tachycardia and tachypnoea were all consistent with high circulating levels of catecholamines; in the presence of high systolic and diastolic blood pressures this is more likely due to anxiety than significant blood loss. However, his usual blood pressure was unknown, and a well maintained haemoglobin and negative faecal occult blood test are poor acute indicators of the extent of blood loss, so the possibility of a substantial bleed had to be considered in the initial management. It is common, as in this case, for the patient to overestimate greatly the quantity of blood lost.

OUTCOME
Intravenous fluids, an H_2-receptor antagonist and an antiemetic were administered and the vomiting settled within a few hours. As is usual in such cases, there was no evidence of further bleeding, nor any subsequent fall in haemoglobin, although the faecal occult blood test became transiently positive.

KEY POINTS
History/Examination
- A history of vomiting unaltered blood beginning *after* the onset of a bout of retching/vomiting is very suggestive of a mucosal tear.

Investigations
- Endoscopy is the only way to make a definitive diagnosis.
- Haemoglobin concentration and faecal occult blood are unreliable early indicators of the extent of blood loss.

Outcome
- This problem is usually self-limiting but substantial blood loss is sometimes encountered.

Richard Thomson (64) Painful foot

CASE HISTORY

Mr Thomson, a retired postman, presented with a 4-day history of painful swelling of the great toe on the right foot. He had found difficulty in wearing shoes and was unable to sleep at night because of pressure from the bedcovers on his foot. He had a past history of ischaemic heart disease, having had a myocardial infarction at age 55 years and again at 59 years. Following these episodes, he had been breathless and was found to have poor left ventricular function with a low cardiac output and persistent cardiac failure. In addition, he had moderately severe chronic obstructive airways disease. He was on regular treatment with a long-acting nitrate, an angiotensin-converting enzyme inhibitor, and inhaled beta agonists and corticosteroids. He used sublingual nitrates intermittently for relief of angina. His daily dose of a loop diuretic had recently been doubled owing to an increase in breathlessness attributed to cardiac failure.

He had a previous history of arthritis affecting his left hip and both hands, and had had several previous episodes of pain in his toe which had been attributed to gout. He had had peptic ulcer sugery when aged 35 years, but had been otherwise well until his first myocardial infarction caused him to take early retirement. He had been a smoker of 35 cigarettes daily until the age of 59 and he drank two or three beers each week. He lived in a ground floor flat with his wife.

EXAMINATION

He was in some distress with pain from his toe, which was hot, red, swollen, tender and rigid (Fig. 45.1). His hands showed swelling, but no tenderness, of the distal interphalangeal joints. His knees were slightly deformed and there was crepitus on flexion. He was apyrexial. His pulse was 90/min and of small volume, and blood pressure was 110/70. The jugular venous pressure was not raised. His apex beat was not palpable and the heart sounds were soft with no added sounds or murmurs. There was no ankle oedema. The chest was hyperinflated, and he was using accessory muscles of respiration. There were bilateral expiratory rhonchi and bilateral basal late inspiratory crackles. Abdominal examination was normal apart from a scar from previous surgery, and there was no neurological abnormality.

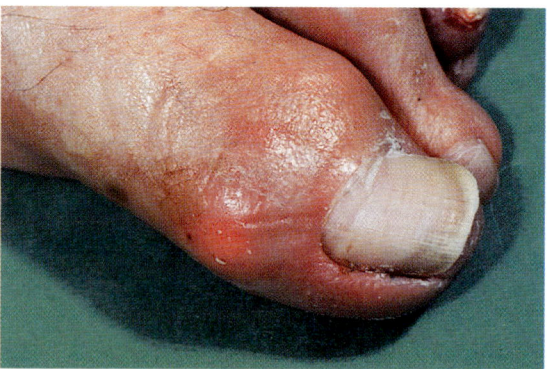

Fig. 45.1 Red swollen toe.

INVESTIGATIONS
Routine investigation results

Urine	SpG 1.015	Pr tr	Glu neg	Ke neg	Blood neg
Serum	Na 137	K 4.5	HCO_3 21	U 26.2	Cr 217
	Alb 43	Bil 12	AAT 22	AP 66	γGT 46
Blood	Hb 145	MCV 92	WCC 12.1	Plt 242	ESR 37

Additional investigations

Radiographs of the right foot revealed no bony abnormality but some soft-tissue swelling around the great toe. Serum uric acid was 0.81 mmol/l (reference range < 0.42).

DIAGNOSIS

The diagnosis, based on the clinical history and elevated serum uric acid, is acute gout, in which the joint inflammation is secondary to deposition of uric acid crystals in the synovial fluid. Gout may occur secondary to an increase in purine turnover, increased urate production or decreased urate excretion. In this case, the most likely precipitating cause is the recent increase in the diuretic dose, which serves to reduce renal clearance of uric acid. The investigations also indicate that Mr Thomson has moderate renal impairment, which is associated with increased serum uric acid and an increased risk of acute gout.

Gout may present as an acute illness involving a single joint or as a chronic arthropathy with deposition of uric acid crystals (monosodium urate monohydrate) in the soft tissues (tophi). Renal calculi may occur as a result of crystallization of uric acid in urine, and thus renal impairment may be the cause or the consequence of gout. The diagnosis of gouty arthropathy may be confirmed by aspiration of the affected joint and examination of the fluid under polarized light microscopy when crystals are seen (Fig. 45.2). Uric acid crystals (negatively birefringent) must be distinguished from calcium pyrophosphate crystals (positively birefringent) which cause pseudogout.

Other causes of painful swelling of a single joint include infection and trauma. Occasionally a generalized arthropathy such as rheumatoid disease may present with single joint involvement.

OUTCOME

He was treated with rest and NSAIDs, and the pain in his toe settled over a period of 4 days. Thereafter, treatment with allopurinol was commenced to prevent further acute attacks of gout. A low dose of allopurinol was used in view of his renal impairment.

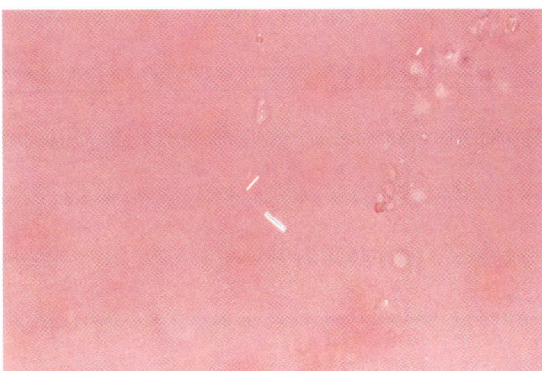

Fig. 45.2
Polarized light microscopy of joint fluid containing crystals.

KEY POINTS

History/Examination
- Acute gout may cause painful swelling of a single joint.
- An increase in diuretic dosage may precipitate acute gout.

Investigations
- A high serum uric acid is usual, but not invariable, in cases of acute gout.

Outcome
- An acute attack of gout should be controlled with anti-inflammatory drugs.
- Allopurinol may be given on a long-term basis to prevent attacks of gout.

David Douglas (54)
Night sweats, tiredness

CASE HISTORY

Mr Douglas, a senior roads supervisor with a local authority, was admitted with a 3-month history of progressive tiredness associated with weight loss of 4 kg. He had also had bouts of sweating, mostly at night, which were occasionally so severe as to cause him to change his pyjamas. He had no cough or sputum production, and no chest pain. He described his appetite as 'fair'. He had had no recent sore throats and had not noted any swollen glands. He had no dysuria or frequency.

In the past he had had pleurisy in his teens, dysentery when with the army overseas, and a vasectomy at age 42 years. His teenage daughter suffered from asthma but there was no other family history of note. Mr Douglas had stopped smoking 15 years earlier; he drank approximately eight units of alcohol per week and had not noted any pain or flushing associated with drinking.

EXAMINATION

On admission he was flushed and pyrexial at 38.1°C. There was no lymphadenopathy, jaundice, finger clubbing, splinter haemorrhages or peripheral oedema. His pulse was 100/min and regular, and blood pressure was 134/82. The jugular venous pressure was not elevated. Examination of the chest and heart was unremarkable. His abdomen was soft and non-tender with no palpable masses or organomegaly, and there were no neurological abnormalities.

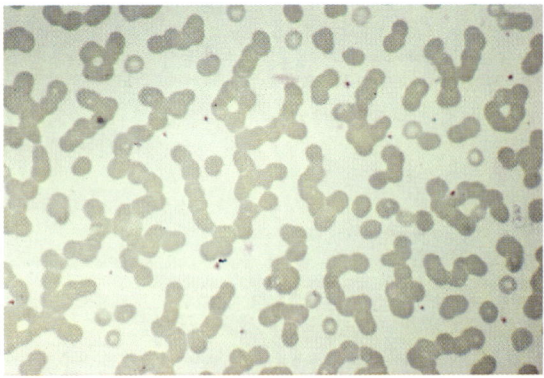

Fig. 46.1
Blood film showing prominent rouleaux formation.

INVESTIGATIONS
Routine investigation results

Urine	SpG 1.025	Pr ++	Glu neg	Ke neg	Blood tr
Serum	Na 136	K 4.6	HCO$_3$ 23	U 7.9	Cr 110
	Alb 32	Bil 18	AAT 32	AP 80	γGT 94
Blood	Hb 116	MCV 86	WCC 14.2	Plt 297	ESR 105

Additional investigations

A blood film showed a normochromic, normocytic anaemia with prominent rouleaux formation (Fig. 46.1). There was a slight neutrophilia, but white blood cell morphology was normal. The chest radiograph was normal. Urine microscopy showed some red cells but no organisms (including acid and alcohol-fast bacteria). Urine and blood cultures showed no growth, and a viral serology screen was negative. The Mantoux test gave a reaction consistent with previous exposure or immunization.

Twenty-four hour urinary protein excretion was 0.65 g (reference range < 0.15) and there was no Bence-Jones protein. Serum calcium was 2.74 mmol/l (2.20–2.60), serum thyroxine 81 nmol/l (70–150) and TSH 0.8 mU/l (0.35–3.30).

DIAGNOSIS

The fever (Fig. 46.2), weight loss, sweats and high ESR could signify underlying infection such as bacterial endocarditis or tuberculosis, a connective tissue disease or a malignancy, especially lymphoma. Unexplained weight loss would suggest malignancy, tuberculosis, hyperthyroidism and diabetes as diagnostic possibilities. The very high ESR would raise the possibilities of myeloma, severe uraemia, cold agglutinins or renal carcinoma.

While most of the investigation results were negative, the presence of haematuria was a crucial clue to the primary pathology. It led to ultrasound scanning of the renal tract, at which a large tumour mass 9 cm in diameter was seen in the upper pole of the left kidney (Fig. 46.3). The presumptive diagnosis of renal

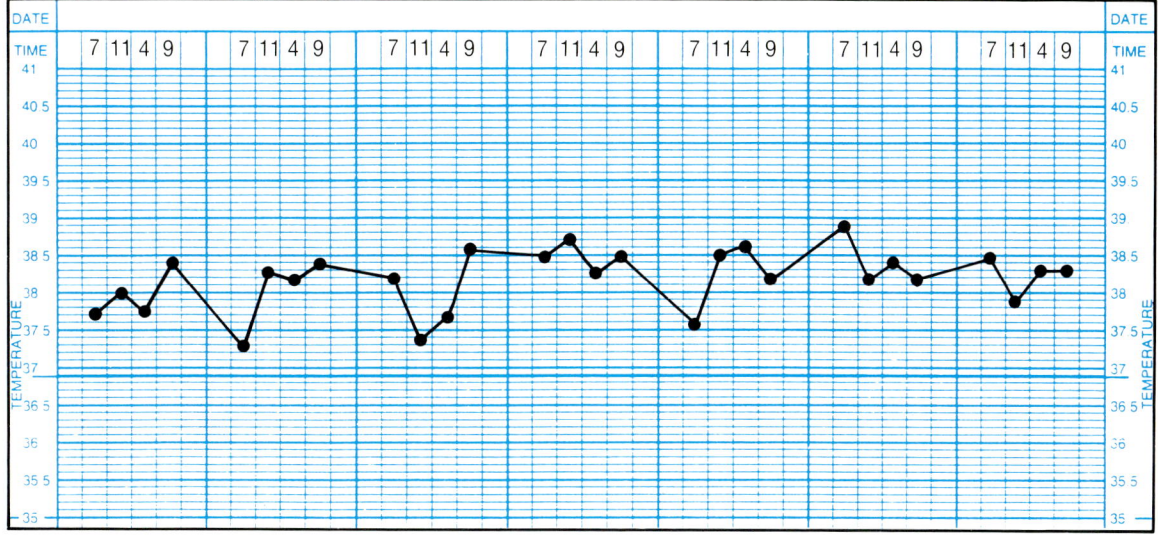

Fig. 46.2
Temperature chart showing persistent variable fever.

carcinoma (hypernephroma) was confirmed by histological examination of the specimen obtained at subsequent left nephrectomy. The serum calcium was high, particularly in view of the low serum albumin (2.74 correcting to 2.94 by adding 0.025 mmol/l per gram of albumin to 40 g/l). This was in keeping with the humoral hypercalcaemia sometimes seen with this type of tumour, which is due to production by the tumour of a substance with parathyroid hormone-like activity. The abnormal liver function tests may have been evidence of hepatic metastases at presentation that were too small to be seen at laparotomy.

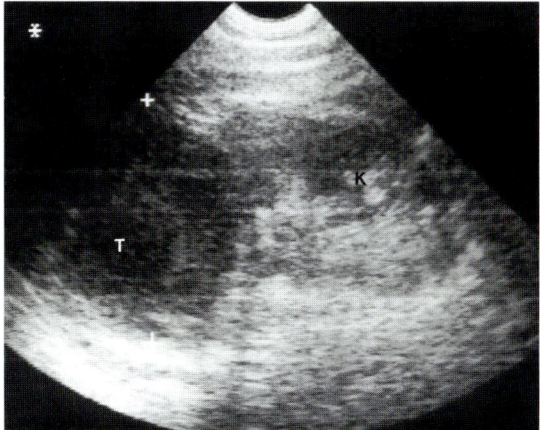

Fig. 46.3
Ultrasound scan section through left kidney demonstrating tumour mass (T) at upper pole of otherwise normal kidney (K). Caliper crosses show maximum tumour diameter of 9 cm.

OUTCOME

Following surgery, the patient had a continuing intermittent fever. He was well enough to go home a week after surgery but remained weak. Six weeks later he was re-admitted with evidence of continued rapid weight loss, fever and vomiting. His renal and hepatic function had deteriorated and he was anaemic and mildly hypercalcaemic. A repeat ultrasound scan showed evidence of multiple hepatic metastases. Mr Douglas died 1 week later of an unusually aggressive renal carcinoma, less than 5 months from his first symptoms.

KEY POINTS

History/Examination
- Renal carcinoma can present with fevers, sweats and weight loss.
- Serious renal pathology is often undetectable on clinical examination.

Investigations
- A finding of microscopic haematuria demands further investigation.
- The ESR is typically very high in patients with renal carcinoma.
- Ultrasound scanning is very useful for demonstrating structural lesions of the kidneys and bladder.

Outcome
- The absence of macroscopic metastatic disease and apparent complete removal of the primary tumour are not necessarily reliable evidence of a cure.

Margaret Errol (76)
Chest pain

CASE HISTORY
Mrs Errol was admitted complaining of sharp right lower chest pain which had begun 24h earlier. The pain had come on suddenly while she was having tea with a friend, and was worse on deep breathing and coughing. She had a dry, unproductive cough and had become breathless even at rest, but had no sputum or haemoptysis.

Her previous medical history included tuberculosis at the age of 30 years, following which she had been told that she had some scarring of the upper lobes of both lungs. She had had a duodenal ulcer, treated medically, at 50 years of age and septic arthritis of the right knee at 63 years. The latter had resulted in severe limitation of movement of the knee joint, and she wore a permanent full-length leg splint. Sixteen days prior to this admission she had undergone a cataract extraction under general anaesthesia. She lived alone, kept a pet cockatiel and was a non-smoker.

EXAMINATION
She was pale, tachypnoeic and pyrexial (38.5°C). Her pulse was 84/min, and blood pressure was 140/60. The second heart sound was loud. Expansion of the chest was limited by pain on the right side and the percussion note was dull at the right base, where a pleural friction rub was audible. Scattered crackles were audible at the left lung base. Abdominal examination was normal. The right leg was immobilized in a splint and there was wasting of the right quadriceps muscle. There was mild oedema of both ankles.

INVESTIGATIONS
Routine investigation results

Urine	SpG 1.005	Pr neg	Glu neg	Ke neg	Blood neg
Serum	Na 133	K 4.4	HCO$_3$ 24	U 5.4	Cr 7
	Alb 34	Bil 4	AAT 32	AP 51	γGT 32
Blood	Hb 122	MCV 93	WCC 10.5	Plt 228	ESR 15

Additional investigations
Arterial blood gases (breathing air) were as follows:

pH	pO$_2$	pCO$_2$	sHCO$_3$
7.51	7.2	3.9	24

An ECG prior to her cataract surgery and another on admission are shown (Fig. 47.1). The chest radiograph on admission was abnormal (Fig. 47.2). The ventilation-perfusion scan confirmed the diagnosis (Fig. 47.3).

DIAGNOSIS
The diagnosis was of pulmonary infarction secondary to deep venous thrombosis.

The history of pain is typical of pleurisy, which is often secondary to underlying lung disease such as pneumonia or infarction. Pulmonary infarction is usually the result of embolization of a blood clot from the deep veins of the lower limb or pelvis. Mrs Errol had two major risk factors for deep vein thrombosis, namely immobility, due to the limited range of movement of her right knee, and recent surgery. Although she did not have clinical signs of lower limb deep vein thrombosis, these are often absent in patients with pulmonary infarction.

The chest radiograph shows opacification in the right lower zone and a right pleural effusion, in addition to patchy shadows in both upper lobes related to her previous tuberculosis. The right lower zone changes are not specific to pulmonary infarction and could occur, for example, in pneumonia. The ventilation-perfusion scan showed matched ventilation and perfusion deficits in the right lower zone, which, like the radiographic changes, are not specific and may occur in pneumonia or segmental lung collapse. However, the diagnosis is confirmed by the unmatched perfusion defect seen in the right upper lobe, which is highly suggestive of pulmonary embolism.

The development of right bundle branch block is a recognized ECG feature of pulmonary embolism. The arterial blood gases show moderate hypoxia, which was due to ventilation-perfusion mismatch. This led to hyperventilation, which resulted in a mild acute respiratory alkalosis.

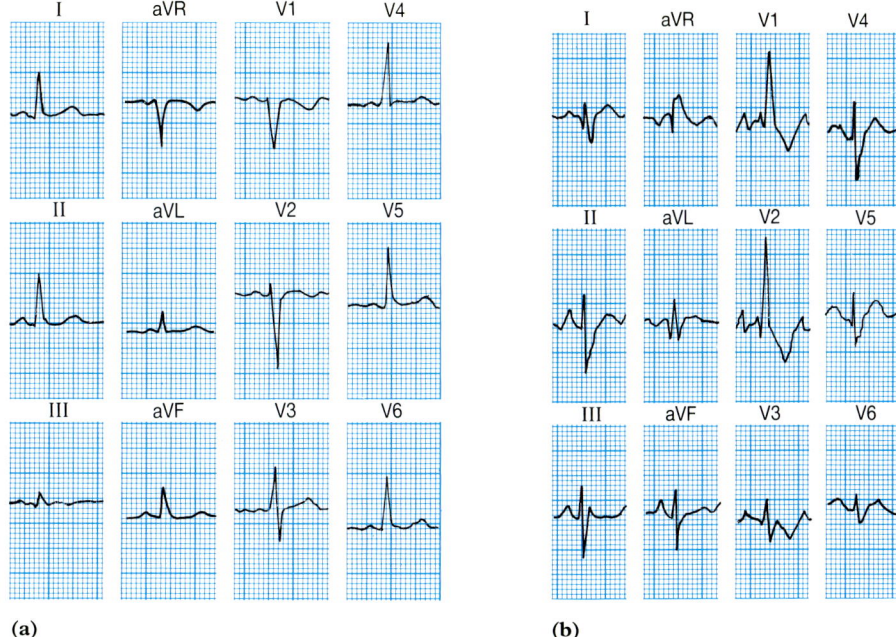

Fig. 47.1
(a) Preoperative ECG showing sinus rhythm and normal QRS complexes. (b) Admission ECG showing right bundle branch block pattern.

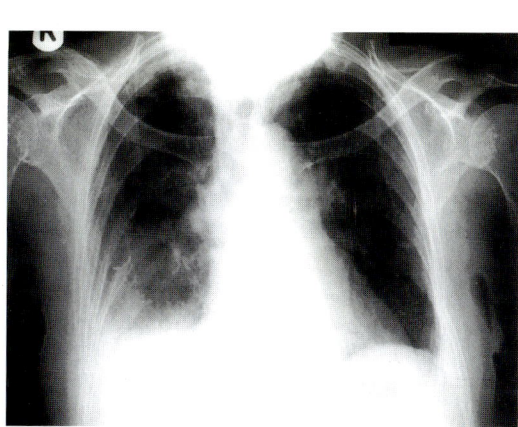

Fig. 47.2
Chest radiograph showing right lower zone opacification with a right pleural effusion. Bilateral patchy apical shadowing is related to fibrosis from previous tuberculosis.

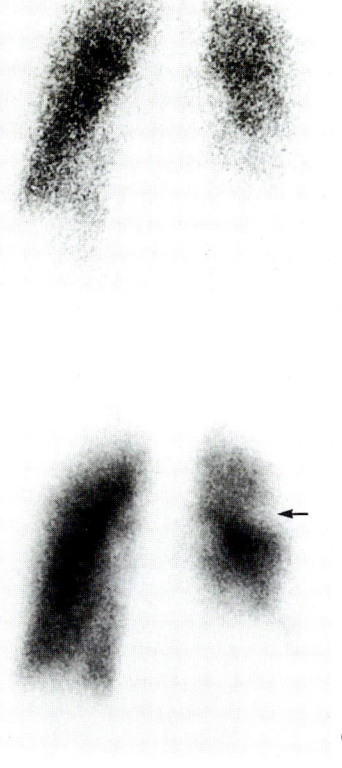

Fig. 47.3
Radioisotopic ventilation (a) and perfusion (b) scans (posterior view) showing matched ventilation and perfusion defects at the right lung apex, due to pulmonary fibrosis, and right lung base, due to pleural effusion. There is an unmatched perfusion defect (arrow) in the right mid-zone, confirming the diagnosis of pulmonary embolism.

OUTCOME

Anticoagulation was administered using heparin and warfarin. The warfarin dose was closely monitored in view of the risks in the elderly, in whom anticoagulation carries a significant morbidity and mortality. However, the risks of treatment must be balanced against the risks of the underlying condition, and in view of her immobilized limb, Mrs Errol was felt to be at high risk of further embolism. She made an uncomplicated recovery.

KEY POINTS

History/Examination
- Consider pulmonary infarction as a cause of pleurisy or haemoptysis.
- Immobility and recent surgery are risk factors for deep vein thrombosis.
- The absence of physical signs does not exclude the diagnosis of deep vein thrombosis.

Investigations
- The development of right bundle branch block is suggestive of pulmonary embolism.
- An unmatched perfusion defect on radioisotopic lung scanning is a diagnostic feature of pulmonary embolism.

Outcome
- Anticoagulant dosage must be monitored carefully.

48 John Wilson (67) Collapse, ? fit

CASE HISTORY
Mr Wilson, a retired gardener, was watching television at home when he suddenly lost consciousness. His wife said that he was 'out cold' for several minutes, and that his right arm had been jerking for part of that time. There was no tongue biting or incontinence. When he regained consciousness, he was confused and drowsy. The ambulancemen who took him to hospital noted that he was weak on his right side and unable to stand unaided. When questioned in hospital approximately 1 h later, he had no recollection of what had happened and denied any weakness. He said he had been having frontal headaches for the previous fortnight, worse during the night. There had been no nausea or vomiting, but some loss of appetite. His wife reported that he had been unusually forgetful in recent weeks, and that he had been smiling more than usual, even at a funeral the previous week.

Past medical history included rheumatic fever in childhood, and a single hospital admission with pneumonia 6 years ago. There was no family history of note. He was not on medication, was a non-smoker and seldom drank alcohol.

EXAMINATION
On arrival in the ward he looked well and was fully conscious and orientated. He appeared inappropriately amused by his circumstances and his speech was a little slurred. He was apyrexial. His pulse was 54/min and regular, and blood pressure was 140/88. The heart sounds were normal, as was examination of the chest and abdomen. There was minimal weakness of his right arm and leg, and the right plantar response was extensor. Tendon jerks were present and equal. There was a suggestion of a right-sided grasp reflex but no demonstrable sensory problem. Examination of the cranial nerves was normal, but fundoscopy revealed a significant abnormality (Fig. 48.1).

INVESTIGATIONS
Routine investigation results

Urine	SpG 1.020	Pr tr	Glu neg	Ke neg	Blood neg
Serum	Na 134	K 3.8	HCO$_3$ 24	U 6.9	Cr 97
	Alb 39	Bil 19	AAT 23	AP 82	γGT 34
Blood	Hb 128	MCV 91	WCC 7.9	Plt 352	ESR 15

Additional investigations
An ECG showed sinus bradycardia with normal complexes. A chest radiograph was normal, but a CT head scan showed a diagnostic abnormality (Fig. 48.2).

DIAGNOSIS
This man had a cerebral tumour as suggested by several elements in the history. He had had headaches, worse on lying down, for some weeks before presentation. His cerebral function had been deteriorating as witnessed by the noticeable failure of recent memory, and his inappropriate euphoria suggested a frontal lobe lesion. Loss of appetite, with or without nausea and vomiting, can be a feature of raised intracranial pressure. His admission was precipitated by a fit with a residual right hemiparesis indicating a left-sided cerebral lesion; the grasp reflex

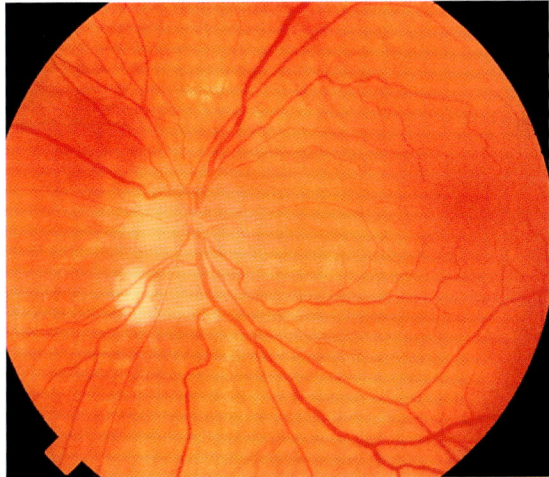

Fig. 48.1
Fundoscopic appearance showing papilloedema.

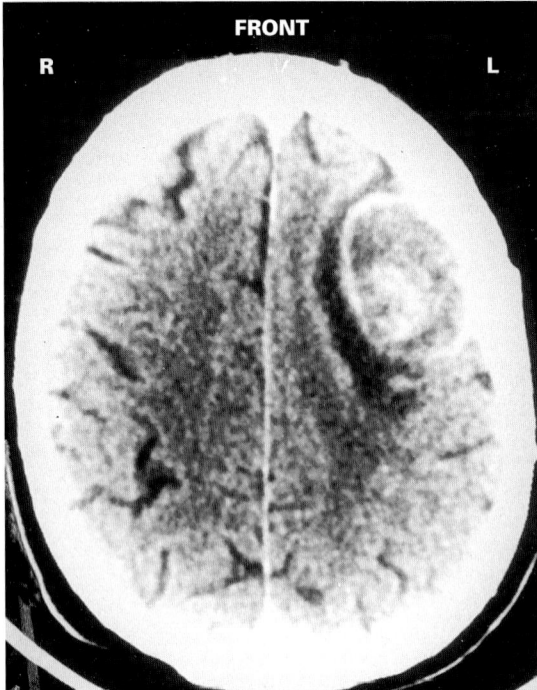

Fig. 48.2
Single transverse CT section through the head showing left frontoparietal tumour.

indicated that this was likely to be frontal. Raised intracranial pressure had led to bradycardia and papilloedema, indicated by blurring of the optic disc margins. The CT head scan showed a 4 cm tumour mass in the left frontoparietal region with some enhancement on injection of contrast medium. There was surrounding cerebral oedema but minimal lateral shift of the ventricular system. Burr hole biopsy examined under frozen section showed the features of a meningioma and the patient proceeded to formal craniotomy and excision of the tumour under the same anaesthetic. A 4 cm x 4 cm x 3 cm mass adherent to the adjacent dura was removed and histology confirmed it to be a meningioma with frequent mitotic figures.

OUTCOME

Mr Wilson was treated with a reducing course of betamethasone in an attempt to reduce the cerebral oedema before, and for 2 weeks after, surgery. He made an excellent recovery and had no neurological deficit by the time of his discharge from hospital on the fifth postoperative day. In view of the numerous mitoses on histology, and uncertainty about completeness of tumour excision, he subsequently proceeded to a 4-week course of radiotherapy to the left posterior frontal region. He remained fit and well 2 years later.

KEY POINTS

History/Examination
- Hemiparesis in an elderly patient is not always due to a cerebrovascular event.
- A short history of persistent headache, which is worse overnight, is suggestive of raised intracranial pressure.
- Focal cerebral disease may give rise to personality change or intellectual impairment.
- Inappropriate euphoria and a grasp reflex are features of frontal lobe disease.

Investigations
- CT head scanning gives useful information about the nature of intracranial structural lesions.
- Biopsy and frozen-section examination may be necessary to confirm the diagnosis and thus the appropriate therapeutic approach to tumour management.

Outcome
- Surgery, plus radiotherapy if appropriate, can produce excellent results in treating meningioma.

Graham Johnson (35)
Breathlessness

CASE HISTORY
Mr Johnson, a musician, had felt generally unwell for 2 months with fatigue, weight loss of about 6 kg and a dry cough. He had seen his general practitioner 4 weeks previously and had been given a 10-day course of erythromycin for a presumed chest infection. Despite the antibiotics he had become gradually more breathless and generally unwell. He was no longer able to perform with his band and as his condition was deteriorating his general practitioner admitted him to hospital.

His previous health had been good. He was single and lived with his parents on a farm, although he travelled abroad frequently in the course of his work. He smoked cigars occasionally and drank three or four pints of beer each week.

EXAMINATION
On admission, he looked well except for some facial folliculitis (Fig. 49.1). He was pyrexial (38.1°C). The fauces were normal but he had moderate oral candidiasis. He had no lymphadenopathy. His pulse was 84/min and regular, and blood pressure was 100/60. His heart sounds were normal. His respiration rate was 23/min, and he had mild central cyanosis. Auscultation of the chest revealed a few inspiratory crackles at both lung bases. The remainder of the examination was normal.

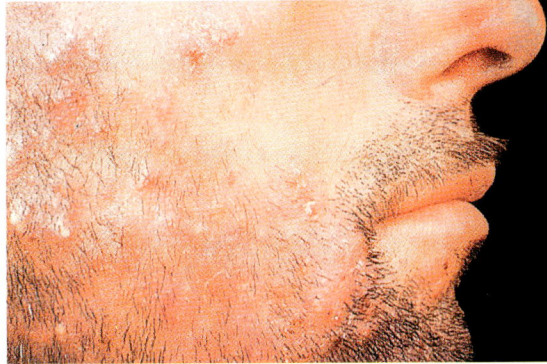

Fig. 49.1
Facial folliculitis.

INVESTIGATIONS
Routine investigation results

Urine	SpG 1.020	Pr neg	Glu neg	Ke neg	Blood neg
Serum	Na 129	K 4.7	HCO_3 24	U 5.8	Cr 96
	Alb 30	Bil 19	AAT 78	AP 80	γGT 34
Blood	Hb 130	MCV 89	WCC 5.5	Plt 178	ESR 64

Additional investigations
A differential white cell count showed 97% neutrophils, 2% lymphocytes and 1% monocytes. Arterial blood gases (breathing air) were as follows:

pH	pO_2	pCO_2	$sHCO_3$
7.41	7.6	4.5	24

The chest radiograph showed abnormalities in both lung fields (Fig. 49.2). Sputum microscopy showed no organisms and culture revealed no growth.

DIAGNOSIS
Mr Johnson's initial history of cough, breathlessness and fever was suggestive of respiratory infection. However, he had failed to respond to antibiotic therapy and initial sputum culture and microscopy were negative. The presence of folliculitis and oral candidiasis and the diffuse radiographic abnormalities alerted the physicians to the possibility that he may be immunocompromised with opportunistic infection. During counselling for a human immunodeficiency virus (HIV) test he told the counsellor that he was homosexual. The HIV test was positive. To obtain further samples for bacteriological examination, bronchoscopy was performed and silver staining of the bronchoalveolar lavage fluid provided the diagnosis (Fig. 49.3).

This patient had *Pneumocystis carinii* pneumonia (PCP) as a result of the acquired immunodeficiency syndrome (AIDS). PCP is the most common

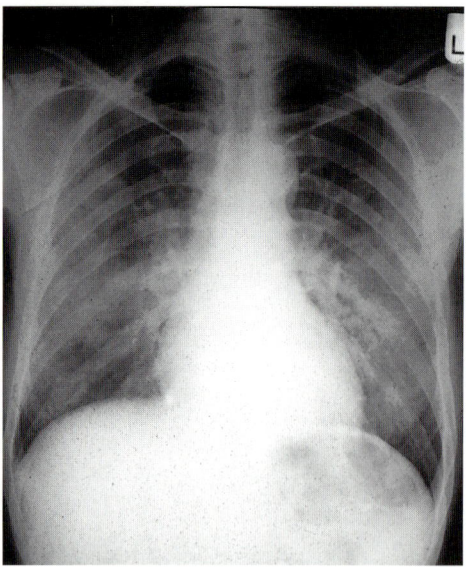

Fig. 49.2
Postero-anterior chest radiograph showing diffuse bilateral reticulonodular shadowing.

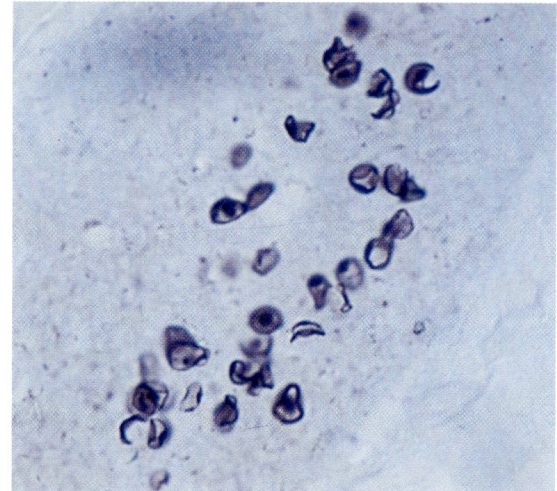

Fig. 49.3
Methenamine silver stain of sputum showing intact cysts with central dot and collapsed cystic forms typical of *Pneumocystis carinii*.

opportunistic infection in AIDS, occurring in up to 80% of individuals infected with HIV. Its course is often insidious and prolonged (weeks to months) and its presence usually indicates profoundly depressed cell-mediated immunity. Hyponatraemia frequently occurs in acute PCP. Good sputum samples are often difficult to obtain in patients with PCP. Sputum, obtained by administering hypertonic nebulized saline to stimulate cough (induced sputum), may be positive for *Pneumocystis* in up to 70% of patients with PCP. Bronchoscopy with bronchoalveolar lavage, peformed in this case, is the 'gold standard' for providing diagnostic specimens.

HIV infection should be suspected in any patient with an atypical illness, regardless of the presence of recognized risk factors such as intravenous drug misuse or homosexuality.

OUTCOME
He was treated successfully with intravenous and oral co-trimoxazole for 21 days. He was discharged on zidovudine (an antiretroviral drug) and prophylactic nebulized pentamidine on a monthly basis.

KEY POINTS

History/Examination
- HIV infection should be suspected in any patient with an atypical illness.

Investigations
- Informed consent is necessary prior to HIV testing in some countries, e.g. the UK.
- Sputum or bronchoalveolar lavage specimens require special stains to diagnose opportunistic infection.

Outcome
- Opportunistic infections in AIDS patients can be successfully treated.

Gerald Millar (73)
Backache, weak legs

CASE HISTORY
Mr Millar, a retired company director, described a 3-month history of pain around the lower chest. The pain was dull and fluctuated in intensity, being worse after prolonged standing. During the 3 weeks prior to admission, he had felt his legs becoming numb and increasingly weak. He had had progressive difficulty in walking, and was unsteady even when standing still. He had no bladder or bowel disturbance.

He had a previous history of ischaemic heart disease and gout. He had formerly had an excessive alcohol intake, amounting to 25 units of alcohol per week, but had abstained from alcohol for the last 2 months. He was taking a variety of drugs, including allopurinol, nifedipine, metoprolol, frusemide and paracetamol. He was a non-smoker, and there was no significant family history.

EXAMINATION
He was obese and plethoric. The cardiovascular and respiratory systems were normal. The liver was palpable 2 cm below the costal margin, the spleen was impalpable and abdominal examination was otherwise normal. Cranial nerve examination was normal. Tone was normal in the arms and increased in both legs. Power of hip flexion was reduced bilaterally, and all muscle groups in the lower limbs were weak. Pin prick sensation was reduced from the level of the costal margin downwards, and proprioception and vibration sense were impaired in both legs. Pain and temperature sensation were normal. Knee jerks and ankle jerks were increased bilaterally. Both plantar responses were extensor.

INVESTIGATIONS
Routine investigation results

Urine	SpG 1.005	Pr neg	Glu neg	Ke neg	Blood neg
Serum	Na 133	K 3.3	HCO₃ 33	U 53	Cr 100
	Alb 48	Bil 9	AAT 43	AP 135	γGT 40
Blood	Hb 105	MCV 92	WCC 7.1	Plt 305	ESR 110

Additional investigations
Serum protein measurements revealed: total protein 79 g/l (reference range 61–76); IgG 9.6 g/l (8–14); IgA 10.2 g/l (0.9–3.5); IgM 0.5 g/l (0.5–2.5).

Serum protein electrophoresis showed a paraprotein band. Urinary Bence-Jones protein was negative.

The dorsal spine radiograph (Fig. 50.1) showed destruction of the vertebral body and pedicle of T6 with narrowing of disc spaces and osteophyte formation. A lumbar myelogram showed an extradural block at the level of T6 (Fig. 50.2). A CT scan of the thoracic spine (Fig. 50.3) showed further detail of the lesion at T6. A bone marrow aspirate showed many plasma cells, including atypical forms (Fig. 50.4). These cells stained for IgA and lambda light chains.

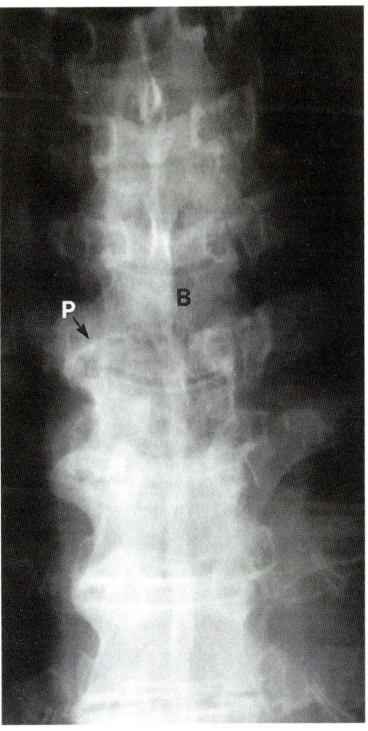

Fig. 50.1
Radiograph of the thoracic spine showing destruction of the vertebral body (B) and pedicle (P) of T6.

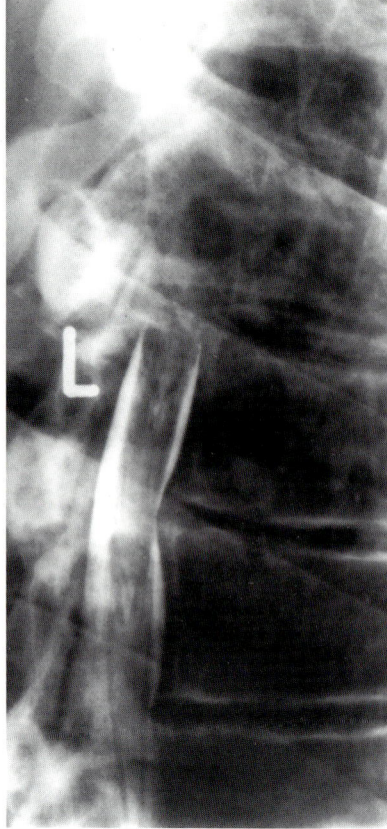

Fig. 50.2
Lateral radiograph of the mid-thoracic region from a myelographic series demonstrating extradural block at the level of T6.

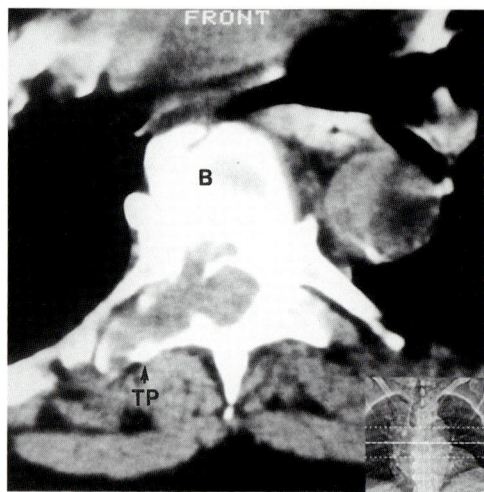

Fig. 50.3
A single transverse CT section through T6 showing lytic destruction of the vertebral body (B) and transverse process (TP). The pedicle has been completely destroyed.

DIAGNOSIS

The lower anterior chest pain was initially attributed to his known ischaemic heart disease. However, the continuous nature of the pain and its relation to posture suggested an alternative diagnosis. The impairment of sensation from the level of the T6/7 dermatome downwards is typical of the presence of spinal cord compression at that level.

Spinal radiographs in this patient showed extensive degenerative change and osteporosis, together with destruction of the vertebral body and pedicle of T6. The CT scan provided more details of the expanding and destructive tumour occupying the body of T6 and extending on the right into the theca. The extradural mass extended up posteriorly to the level of the body of T5 and down to the upper margin of T7.

The elevated total plasma protein and the high level of IgA with paraprotein band were suggestive of the diagnosis of myeloma, which was confirmed by the bone marrow findings. The diagnosis was therefore multiple myeloma (IgA type) with spinal cord compression at the T6 level resulting from a localized bony myelomatous deposit.

Haematological features on the routine investigations indicating a possible diagnosis of myeloma are the anaemia and the high ESR. Bence-Jones proteinuria was absent in this patient, but occurs in about 40% of patients who have IgA myeloma. Mild elevation of the alkaline phosphatase may be a pointer to bony destruction, but in this patient, the

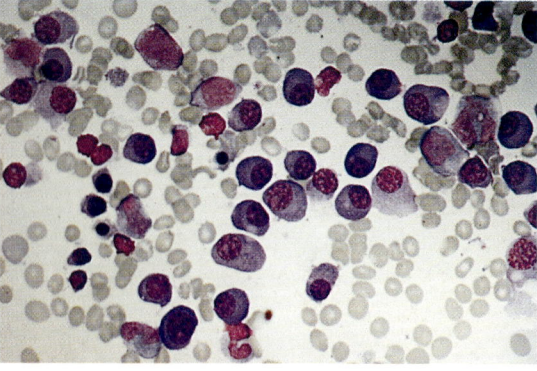

Fig. 50.4
Romanowsky stain of bone marrow aspirate showing plasma cells, including atypical forms.

alkaline phosphatase could also be of liver origin and related to alcoholic liver disease. The source of the elevated blood alkaline phosphatase could be determined by examining isoenzymes.

In addition to expanding tumour deposits, which are relatively unusual, myeloma more often produces osteolytic bony lesions which are visible on radiology. These lesions may not be detected by isotope bone scanning, which is based on detection of osteoblastic activity.

OUTCOME

Mr Millar underwent urgent decompression laminectomy with partial removal of the localized tumour at T6. Histology confirmed the lesion to be a myelomatous deposit. Complete excision was not possible, and surgery was followed by radiotherapy. He made a good, though incomplete, recovery and was able to walk with a rather spastic gait. His sensory signs improved. In view of the positive bone marrow examination confirming disseminated myeloma, he commenced chemotherapy.

KEY POINTS

History/Examination
- History and examination findings suggestive of spinal cord compression require urgent investigation and treatment.

Investigations
- Myeloma should always be considered in the differential diagnosis of a very high ESR.
- CT scanning is a sensitive method for detecting lesions involving the axial skeleton.
- Bence-Jones proteinuria suggests myeloma when positive, but does not exclude myeloma when negative.

Outcome
- Local treatment is appropriate for the local effects of a myelomatous deposit (plasmacytoma).
- Systemic treatment is necessary in disseminated myelomatosis.

Section 2
Self-assessment exercises

This section includes a number of self-assessment exercises based exclusively on the content of the book, such that the correct answer is given by referencing the chapter or chapters in which the relevant information is given or explained. The exercises are intended to subserve a number of separate functions for the reader. They allow assessment of the extent to which factual material has been retained, they provide a guide on the need for revision of pertinent chapters, and in some instances they emphasize similarities and contrasts in the presentation and investigation of different conditions. Since the majority of readers are likely to be prospective examinees, useful practice is also provided.

There are two basic formats employed, both using a simple true/false approach. The first sets of questions consist of a 'stem' statement with five related parts each requiring a true or false response; the stems are roughly organized in order into questions relating to history, followed by examination, followed by investigation. There then follows a series of five composite quizzes each comprising 12 individual true/false questions. The answers to the true/false sets and to Quizzes 1–5 are given at the end of each self-assessment section.

MCQs

1. Sudden loss of consciousness can be a feature of:-

a) Stokes-Adams attacks
b) Paracetamol poisoning
c) Hyperosmolar non-ketotic diabetic state
d) Epilepsy
e) Acute gastrointestinal haemorrhage

2. A history of smoking is associated with:-

a) Ischaemic heart disease
b) Emphysema
c) Carcinoma of the oesophagus
d) Pericarditis
e) Bronchial carcinoma

3. Recent weight loss may suggest a diagnosis of:-

a) Thyrotoxicosis
b) Neoplastic disease
c) Acquired immunodeficiency syndrome
d) Pulmonary tuberculosis
e) Nephrotic syndrome

4. Pleuritic chest pain is common in:-

a) Pneumothorax
b) Pulmonary thromboembolism
c) Acute myocardial infarction
d) Oesophageal carcinoma
e) Lobar pneumonia

5. A history of excessive sweating is often found in:-

a) Colonic carcinoma
b) Lymphoma
c) Pulmonary tuberculosis
d) Renal carcinoma
e) Infective endocarditis

6. Acute severe abdominal pain typically occurs in:-

a) Ascending cholangitis
b) Leaking aortic aneurysm
c) Acute pancreatitis
d) Infective hepatitis
e) Bleeding duodenal ulcer

7. Diarrhoea often occurs with:-

a) Hypercalcaemia
b) Salmonella food poisoning
c) Thyrotoxicosis
d) Ulcerative colitis
e) Gastric mucosal tear

8. Severe headache can suggest a diagnosis of:-

a) Subarachnoid haemorrhage
b) Bacterial meningitis
c) Subdural haematoma
d) Postural hypotension
e) Cerebral tumour

9. Increasing dyspnoea of effort is a symptom of:-

a) Hepatic metastases
b) Viral pericarditis
c) Anaemia
d) Diabetic ketoacidosis
e) Cardiac failure

10. Development of a skin rash is typical in:-

a) Salmonella food poisoning
b) Meningococcal septicaemia
c) Pernicious anaemia
d) Shingles
e) Ampicillin-treated infectious mononucleosis

11. Jaundice is usually present in cases of:-

a) Acute pancreatitis
b) Viral hepatitis
c) Hypothermia
d) Alcoholic cirrhosis
e) Cholangitis

12. **Bradycardia is a feature of:-**

a) Thyrotoxicosis
b) Raised intracranial pressure
c) Hypothermia
d) Metabolic acidosis
e) Complete heart block

13. **Pyrexia is a common feature of:-**

a) Lymphoma
b) Renal carcinoma
c) Acute ulcerative colitis
d) Meningitis
e) Salmonellosis

14. **Haematuria is a common finding in:-**

a) Nephrotic syndrome
b) Renal calculus disease
c) Renal carcinoma
d) Infectious mononucleosis
e) Infective endocarditis

15. **Hypoalbuminaemia is likely to be found in:-**

a) Alcoholic cirrhosis
b) Nephrotic syndrome
c) Infective endocarditis
d) Salmonella gastroenteritis
e) Inflammatory bowel disease

16. **A low serum bicarbonate concentration is a feature of:-**

a) Chronic obstructive airways disease
b) Tissue hypoperfusion
c) Renal failure
d) Erosive gastritis
e) Diabetic ketoacidosis

17. **A low haemoglobin concentration is a typical feature of:-**

a) Acute gastrointestinal blood loss
b) Chronic gastrointestinal blood loss
c) Chronic renal failure
d) Acute bacterial infection
e) Chronic obstructive airways disease

18. **A very high ESR is found in:-**

a) Myeloma
b) Renal carcinoma
c) Primary cerebral tumour
d) Hypothermia
e) Pulmonary thromboembolism

19. **Elevation of serum alkaline phosphatase is usually found in:-**

a) Biliary tract obstruction
b) Acute gout
c) Primary colonic carcinoma
d) Metastatic liver disease
e) Nephrotic syndrome

20. **Hyperkalaemia is often found in the following:-**

a) Hypothermia
b) Diarrhoea
c) Diabetic ketoacidosis
d) Hyperosmolar non-ketotic diabetic state
e) Overdiuresis

21. **An elevated serum aspartate aminotransferase is found in cases of:-**

a) Hepatocellular disease
b) Viral pericarditis
c) Ruptured aortic aneurysm
d) Myocardial infarction
e) Stokes-Adams attacks

22. **An abnormally low serum urea concentration is typical of:-**

a) Acute upper gastrointestinal bleeding
b) Nephrotic syndrome
e) Hyperosmolar non-ketotic diabetic state
d) Hepatic cirrhosis
e) Gout

23. **Red cell macrocytosis is found in:-**

a) Alcohol excess
b) Hyperthyroidism
c) Pernicious anaemia
d) Inflammatory bowel disease
e) Chronic renal failure

24. An elevated arterial pCO$_2$ is a feature of:-

a) Mild to moderate asthma
b) Pulmonary infarction
c) Diabetic ketoacidosis
d) Acute pancreatitis
e) Chronic obstructive airways disease

25. Hypercalcaemia is a recognized feature of:-

a) Acute pancreatitis
b) Hypoalbuminaemia
c) Squamous carcinoma of the bronchus
d) Renal carcinoma
e) Pernicious anaemia

26. Electrocardiography is useful in the diagnosis of:-

a) Complete heart block
b) Acute myocardial infarction
c) Pericarditis
d) Pulmonary thromboembolism
e) Infective endocarditis

27. Ultrasound scanning is useful in the diagnosis of the following cardiovascular disorders:-

a) Aortic aneurysm
b) Infective endocarditis
c) Acute myocardial infarction
d) Pericardial effusion
e) Cerebral thrombosis

28. Abdominal ultrasound scanning can be useful in demonstrating the presence of:-

a) Cholelithiasis
b) Colonic carcinoma
c) Nephrotic syndrome
d) Renal carcinoma
e) Bladder outlet obstruction

MCQ answers

The numbers in parentheses which follow the answers refer to the case histories.

1. a) T (15)
   b) F (20)
   c) F (13)
   d) T (17, 43, 48)
   e) T (19)

2. a) T (10, 34)
   b) T (5)
   c) T (14)
   d) F (27)
   e) T (9, 37)

3. a) T (1)
   b) T (9, 22, 25, 32, 37, 46)
   c) T (49)
   d) T (30)
   e) F (40)

4. a) T (35)
   b) T (47)
   c) F (10)
   d) F (14)
   e) T (39)

5. a) F (11)
   b) T (32)
   c) T (30)
   d) T (46)
   e) T (3)

6. a) T (36)
   b) T (7)
   c) T (38)
   d) F (18)
   e) F (19)

7. a) F (37)
   b) T (6)
   c) T (1)
   d) T (24)
   e) F (44)

8. a) T (4)
   b) T (33)
   c) T (43)
   d) F (31)
   e) T (48)

9. a) F (22)
   b) F (27)
   c) T (11, 16, 26)
   d) F (28)
   e) T (1, 34)

10. a) F (6)
    b) T (33)
    c) F (26)
    d) T (42)
    e) T (12)

11. a) F (38)
    b) T (18)
    c) F (41)
    d) F (2)
    e) T (36)

12. a) F (1)
    b) T (43, 48)
    c) T (41)
    d) F (13, 28)
    e) T (15)

13. a) T (32)
    b) T (46)
    c) T (24)
    d) T (33)
    e) T (6)

14. a) F (40)
    b) T (16)
    c) T (46)
    d) F (12)
    e) T (3)

15. a) T (2)
    b) T (40)
    c) T (3)
    d) F (6)
    e) T (24)

16. a) F (5)
    b) T (13, 38)
    c) T (16, 31, 34)
    d) F (8)
    e) T (28)

17. a) F (19, 44)
    b) T (8, 11, 24)
    c) T (16, 34)
    d) F (6, 21, 33, 39)
    e) F (5)

18. a) T (50)
    b) T (46)
    c) F (48)
    d) F (41)
    e) F (47)

19. a) T (36)
    b) F (45)
    c) F (11)
    d) T (22)
    e) F (40)

20. a) T (41)
    b) F (6, 24)
    c) T (28)
    d) T (13)
    e) T (31)

21. a) T (12, 18, 20, 22)
    b) F (27)
    c) F (7)
    d) T (10)
    e) F (15)

22. a) F (8, 19, 44)
    b) F (40)
    c) F (13)
    d) T (2)
    e) F (45)

23. a) T (2)
    b) F (1)
    c) T (26)
    d) F (24)
    e) F (16, 34)

24. a) F (23)
    b) F (47)
    c) F (28)
    d) F (38)
    e) T (5)

25. a) F (38)
    b) F (9, 25)
    c) T (37)
    d) T (46)
    e) F (26)

26. a) T (15)
    b) T (10)
    c) T (27)
    d) T (47)
    e) F (3)

27. a) T (7)
    b) T (3)
    c) F (10)
    d) T (27)
    e) F (29)

28. a) T (36)
    b) F (11)
    c) F (40)
    d) T (46)
    e) T (34)

Quiz questions

Quiz 1

Are the following statements true or false?

1. Plantar responses are usually flexor in thoracic spinal cord compression

2. A pericardial friction rub is typically affected by posture

3. Sputum cytology may yield a diagnosis of bronchial carcinoma

4. Lactic acidosis is always a fatal condition

5. Aphthous ulceration is a feature of inflammatory bowel disease

6. Inequality of femoral pulses suggests the presence of aortic dissection

7. The presence of pus cells and 10^4 organisms /mm³ is said to be diagnostic of urinary tract infection

8. On a normal postero-anterior chest radiograph the cardiothoracic ratio is normally 50–67%

9. The jugular venous pressure is usually raised in nephrotic syndrome

10. The presence of gallstones is often an incidental finding on an abdominal ultrasound scan

11. Bilirubinuria is usually found in obstructive jaundice

12. Thyroid size is a useful clinical indicator of thyroid function

Quiz 2

Are the following statements true or false?

1. In cases of substantial gastrointestinal bleeding, bowel sounds are typically infrequent

2. Cardiac failure is a common presentation of thyrotoxicosis in the elderly

3. Neck stiffness usually develops suddenly after subarachnoid haemorrhage

4. Treatment of pernicious anaemia with vitamin B_{12} may cause hypokalaemia

5. Bence-Jones proteinuria is almost always present in myeloma

6. *Salmonella typhi* is a common cause of bacterial gastroenteritis

7. Hemiparesis following a grand mal convulsion often resolves completely

8. Serum bilirubin may be normal in hepatitis A infection

9. Urinary tract infection may be asymptomatic

10. In a severe asthma attack the pulse pressure falls during expiration

11. Dysphasia is a disorder of speech articulation

12. Hypocalcaemia is a poor prognostic indicator in acute pancreatitis

Quiz 3

Are the following statements true or false?

1. Pleural effusion is a recognized feature of pulmonary infarction

2. On the ECG, ST segment depression suggests a diagnosis of pericarditis

3. Facial weakness sparing the upper part of the face occurs with an upper motor neurone facial nerve lesion

4. Thrombolytic therapy in acute myocardial infarction may limit infarct size

5. Leuconychia suggests the presence of iron deficiency

6. The Monospot test is always positive in infectious mononucleosis

7. Aspirin may induce gastrointestinal haemorrhage in the absence of a history of peptic ulcer disease

8. A flapping tremor is a feature of hypoxia

9. Following haematemesis, a tachycardia always signifies substantial blood loss

10. Alcoholic cirrhosis is associated with an increased incidence of hepatocellular carcinoma

11. Acidosis in diabetes is always due to accumulation of ketone bodies

12. Chronic renal failure is associated with anorexia

Quiz 4

Are the following statements true or false?

1. Pneumothorax must always be treated by insertion of a chest drain

2. The ingestion of alcohol predisposes to hypothermia

3. Serum amylase is usually markedly elevated in acute pancreatitis

4. Diuretic therapy increases the excretion of uric acid

5. Candidiasis often occurs in immunosuppressed patients

6. Plasma osmolality is typically normal in the syndrome of inappropriate antidiuretic hormone secretion

7. Acute abdominal pain can be a presenting feature in diabetic ketoacidosis

8. Serum cholesterol is usually low in nephrotic syndrome

9. Hypercalcaemia may give rise to thirst and polyuria

10. The presence of an arcus senilis is usually of clinical significance

11. Macular rash is the first feature of shingles

12. P pulmonale is an electrocardiographic feature of chronic obstructive airways disease

Quiz 5

Are the following statements true or false?

1. Carcinoma of the head of pancreas commonly presents with right upper quadrant pain and jaundice

2. Electrocardiographic J waves are found in pulmonary embolism

3. Elevation of total serum protein is often found in myeloma

4. Hyporeflexia excludes the presence of an upper motor neurone lesion

5. Structural abnormalities predispose to infection in the urinary tract

6. Jaundice in pernicious anaemia is due to associated hepatitis

7. Lymphopenia is a feature of acquired immunodeficiency syndrome

8. Matched defects on a ventilation/perfusion lung scan confirm a diagnosis of pulmonary embolism

9. Hyperventilation may give rise to metabolic acidosis

10. Hypertrophic pulmonary osteoarthropathy is an infrequent complication of bronchial carcinoma

11. Morning headache is a feature of raised intracranial pressure

12. Total serum thyroxine concentration is reduced in hypoproteinaemic states

Quiz answers

The numbers in parentheses which follow the answers refer to the case histories.

Quiz 1

1. F (50)
2. T (27)
3. T (9)
4. F (13)
5. T (24)
6. T (7)
7. F (16)
8. F (13)
9. F (40)
10. T (25)
11. T (22, 36)
12. F (1)

Quiz 3

1. T (47)
2. F (27)
3. T (29)
4. T (10)
5. F (2, 11)
6. F (12)
7. T (8)
8. F (5)
9. F (44)
10. T (2)
11. F (13)
12. T (16)

Quiz 5

1. F (36)
2. F (41, 47)
3. T (50)
4. F (29)
5. T (21)
6. F (26)
7. T (49)
8. F (47)
9. F (20)
10. T (9)
11. T (43, 48)
12. T (40)

Quiz 2

1. F (8, 19)
2. T (1)
3. F (4)
4. T (26)
5. F (50)
6. F (6)
7. T (17)
8. T (18)
9. T (21)
10. F (23)
11. F (4)
12. T (38)

Quiz 4

1. F (35)
2. T (41)
3. T (38, 41)
4. F (45)
5. T (49)
6. F (31)
7. T (28)
8. F (40)
9. T (37)
10. F (34)
11. F (42)
12. T (5)

Index

Abdominal distension, 4, 84
   mass, pulsatile, 17
Acidosis, lactic, 32
   metabolic, 31, 63, 85, 91
   respiratory, 13
AIDS, 107
Airways disease, chronic
     obstructive, 13, 66, 68, 98
Alcohol, excess intake, 4, 20, 67, 84, 94, 96
   withdrawal, 95
Alkaline phosphatase, isoenzymes, 111
Alkalosis, respiratory 46, 102
Alpha-fetoprotein, 5
Amylase, serum, 62, 80, 84, 90
Anaemia, macrocytic, 58
   microcytic, 20, 27, 54
   normocytic, 8, 23, 37, 49, 72, 75, 92, 100, 109
   pernicious, 58
Aneurysm, aortic, 17
   berry, 10
   cerebral, 10
Angina, 17, 20, 25, 98
Angiography, carotid, 10
Ankle jerks, absent, 59
Antibody, anti-mitochondrial, 5
   anti-nuclear, 5
   anti-smooth muscle, 5
   anti-thyroid, 2
   gastric parietal cell, 58
   intrinsic factor, 58
Antistreptolysin-O, 30
Aorta, calcified, 17, 18, 76
   dissection, 17, 25
Aortic regurgitation, 8
Aortic valve, bicuspid, 8
Apraxia, constructional, 5
Arrhythmia, cardiac, 36, 91
Arthritis, 98, 102
Ascites, 5, 89
Asthma, 51
Atrophy, testicular, 4

Bacteraemia, 8, 81, 85
Bence-Jones proteinuria, 100, 109
Biliary obstruction, 50, 81
Bilirubinuria, 49, 80
Biopsy, bone marrow, 93, 109
   brain, 106
   bronchial, 22, 83
   liver, 5
   lymph node, 71
   rectal, 54
   renal, 89

Blackouts, 35, 39, 94, 105
Bladder, distension, 75
Blood film, 37, 58, 93, 100
   gases, arterial, 13, 31, 46, 51, 52, 62, 66, 78, 84, 86, 102, 107
Bowel sounds, absent, 84
   active, 15, 20, 43, 54
Bradycardia, 35, 90
Breath sounds, abnormal, 2, 4, 7, 13, 22, 33, 49, 51, 66, 68, 75, 78, 82, 84, 86, 90, 98, 102, 107
Breathlessness, 2, 4, 7, 12, 22, 27, 31, 37, 51, 58, 62, 66, 68, 75, 78, 88, 98, 102, 107
Bronchoalveolar lavage, 107
Bronchoscopy, 22, 82, 107
Bruising, 58
Bruit, carotid, 17
   femoral, 17
Burr cells, 37

C-reactive protein, 8
Calculi, biliary, 56, 80
   renal, 37, 99
Campylobacter jejuni, 15
Candidiasis, oral, 107
Carcinoma, breast, 49
   bronchial, 23, 82
   colonic, 28
   hepatocellular, 5
   oesophageal, 34
   pancreatic, 57, 81
   prostate, 76
   renal, 100
Cardiomegaly, 31, 68, 75
   radiographic definition, 32
Cardiothoracic ratio, 32
Carpopedal spasm, 45
Catecholamines, 97
Cavitation, pulmonary, 67
Cerebral abscess, 74
Cerebrospinal fluid, 10, 39, 73
Cerebrovascular accident, 65
Chest, hyperinflation, 13, 33, 51, 98
Chlamydia pneumoniae, 87
Cholangitis, acute, 81, 85
Cholestasis, 81
Cirrhosis, alcoholic, 5
   primary biliary, 5
Claudication, intermittent, 17
Clotting studies, 5, 46
Cold agglutinins, 100
Collapse, 17, 20, 39, 43, 64, 94, 105
Colonoscopy, 55
Coma, hepatic, 5

Complement, serum, 88
Confusion, 31, 84, 86, 105
Connective tissue disease, 100
Consolidation, pulmonary, 22, 87
Constipation, 82
Copper, serum, 5
Cor pulmonale, 13
Corneal arcus senilis, 75
Cortisol, plasma, 68
Cough, productive 12, 66
   unproductive, 2, 22, 31, 51, 73, 86, 102, 107
Coxsackie virus, 61
Creatine kinase, 25
Crystals, synovial fluid, 99
Culture, blood, 8, 15, 80, 87
Culture, sputum, 13, 67
   stool, 15, 54
   urine, 37, 47
Cyanosis, central, 12, 51, 66, 86, 107
   peripheral, 31, 90
Cytology, sputum, 22
Cytomegalovirus, 30

Dehydration, 15, 29, 31, 34, 63, 80, 83
Diabetes insipidus, 63, 83
   mellitus, 25, 63, 83, 100
Diarrhoea, 15, 43, 54, 56
Dizziness, postural, 68
Drowsiness, 9, 12, 25, 31, 39, 62, 90, 94, 105
Drug, adverse reaction, 30
   compliance, 69, 89
Dysphagia, 33, 34
Dysphasia, 10, 65
Dysuria, 47

Echocardiography, 8, 61
Eczema, 51
Effusion, pericardial, 61
   pleural, 3, 5, 85, 88, 102
Electrocardiograph, T inversion, 26, 76
   atrial fibrillation, 3
   complete heart block, 35
   hypothermia, 91
   left ventricular hypertrophy, 32
   P pulmonale, 13
   pacing spikes, 36
   Q waves, 26, 76
   right axis deviation, 13
   right bundle branch block, 103
   ST elevation, 26, 60
   ventricular fibrillation, 91

Electroencephalogram (EEG), 40
Embolism, pulmonary, 25, 102
Emphysema, 14, 66
Endocarditis, bacterial, 8, 100
Endoscopic retrograde cholangiopancreatography (ERCP), 57, 80
Endoscopy, upper gastrointestinal, 20, 43, 96
Enzymes, cardiac, 25, 26
Epilepsy, 40, 95
Epstein-Barr virus, 30, 72
Erythema, palmar, 4
Erythrocytosis, secondary, 13
Escherichia coli, 37, 47, 80
ESR, elevated, 4, 7, 13, 23, 31, 33, 47, 49, 54, 58, 60, 66, 72, 73, 80, 82, 84, 86, 92, 100, 107, 109

Faecal occult blood, 20, 27, 33, 43
Failure, cardiac, 3, 59, 68, 77, 98
  renal, acute, 18, 85
  renal, chronic, 38, 76, 83, 99
  right heart, 13
  ventilatory, 13
Fauces, oedematous, 29
Ferritin, serum, 5, 28
Fever, 7, 12, 15, 29, 39, 41, 47, 54, 62, 66, 71, 73, 80, 84, 86, 93, 100, 102, 107
Fibrillation, atrial, 3
Fibrillation, ventricular, 91
Fibrosis, post-irradiation, 50
Fingers, clubbing, 22, 82
  tar staining, 17, 22, 82, 84
Fit, 39, 94, 105
Folate levels, 58
Folliculitis, facial, 107

Gastritis, erosive, 20, 96
Gastroenteritis, 15
Glandular fever, 30
Glomerulonephritis, 89
Glossitis, 58
Glycosuria, 31, 62, 84
Goitre, toxic multinodular, 3
Gout, 98
Grand mal fits, 40, 95
Grasp reflex, 105
Graves' disease, 3
Grey-Turner's sign, 84
Gynaecomastia, 4

Haematemesis, 20
Haematocrit, raised, 13
Haematuria, 7, 18, 37, 47, 100
Haemolysis, 59
Haemophilus influenzae, 13
Haemoptysis, 23
Haemorrhage, cerebral, 65
  gastrointestinal, 28, 43, 54
  retinal, 25
  splinter, 8
  subarachnoid, 9
  subhyaloid, 9
Hard exudates, retinal, 25
Headache, 9, 39, 47, 60, 64, 73, 86, 94, 105
Heart block, complete, 35
Hemiparesis, 10, 39, 64, 94, 105
Hepatitis, 30, 42
  B surface antigen, 5, 41
  chronic active, 5
Hepatomegaly, 4, 29, 41, 49, 71, 77
Herpes labialis, 86
  zoster, 92
HIV, 30, 72, 107
Hodgkin's lymphoma, 72
Hydronephrosis, 38, 75
Hypercalcaemia, 63, 82, 100
Hypercapnia, 13, 53
Hypercholesterolaemia, 88
Hyperglycaemia, 31, 63, 84
Hyperkalaemia, 91
Hyperlipidaemia, 26, 77, 88
Hypernephroma, 101
Hyperosmolarity, serum, 31
Hypertension, portal, 5
  pulmonary, 22
  systemic, 22, 31, 64
Hyperthyroidism, 3, 23, 28, 100
Hypertrophy, left ventricular, 32
Hyperventilation, 32, 46, 63, 102
Hypoalbuminaemia, 4, 23, 33, 49, 54, 56, 86, 88, 107
  mechanisms, 89
Hypocalcaemia, 23, 57, 84
Hypogammaglobulinaemia, 93
Hypoglycaemia, 40, 91
Hypokalaemia, 63, 83
Hyponatraemia, 68, 107
Hypotension, 17, 20, 31, 62, 84, 90
  postural, 35, 68, 88
Hypothermia, 90
Hypothyroidism, 56
Hypoxia, 13, 31, 66, 78, 84, 87
  tissue, 32, 85, 102

Iatrogenic disease, 70
Immunoglobulin E, 51
  serum, 93, 109
Indigestion, 20
Infarction, myocardial, 18, 25
  pulmonary, 102
Infection, chest, 31, 107
  opportunistic, 93, 107
  throat, 29
Infectious mononucleosis, 30, 42
Injury, head, 39, 64
  self-inflicted, 45
Iron, serum, 28
Ischaemia, myocardial, 25, 110

Jaundice, 41, 46, 49, 57, 58, 80
Joint aspiration, 99

Kernig's sign, 73

Ketoacidosis, diabetic, 63
Ketonuria, 15, 33, 45, 47, 62, 73, 80, 90, 92
Kidney, duplex, 47
Klebsiella pneumoniae, 87
Koilonychia, 27
Kussmaul respiration, 63

Lactate dehydrogenase, 25
  serum, 31
Laparotomy, diagnostic, 57
Legionella pneumophila, 87
Leucocytosis, 7, 13, 15, 31, 39, 45, 47, 51, 62, 72, 73, 80, 84, 86, 92, 100
Leuconychia, 4
Leukaemia, chronic lymphocytic, 93
Liver, abnormal function tests, 4, 30, 41, 45, 46, 49, 66, 76, 80, 84, 86, 92, 94, 100, 109
Lumbar puncture, 10, 39, 73
Lymphadenopathy, axillary, 29, 92
  cervical, 29, 62, 66, 71
  hilar, 72
  inguinal, 71, 92
  mediastinal, 72
  retroperitoneal, 72
Lymphocytosis, 30, 93
Lymphoma, 72, 100

Macrocytosis, 5, 58, 66, 94
Malabsorption, 57
  vitamin B_{12}, 59
Mantoux test, 100
Mastectomy, 49
Melaena, 43
Meningeal irritation, 10
Meningioma, 106
Meningitis, 74
Meningococcus, 74
Metastases, intrahepatic, 49, 101
Monospot test, 30
Mucosal tear, oesophageal, 96
Murmur, aortic sclerotic, 3
  changing, 8
  early diastolic, 7
  flow, 28, 38
  systolic, 2, 27, 37, 58
Muscle, wasting, 4, 102
Mycobacterium tuberculosis, 67
Mycoplasma pneumoniae, 87
Myelogram, lumbar, 109
Myeloma, 100, 110
  bone marrow appearances, 109

Nausea, 17, 20, 25, 41, 45, 62, 75, 80, 96
Nephropathy, minimal change, 89
Nephrotic syndrome, 89
Neuralgia, post-herpetic, 93
Neutrophils, hypersegmented, 58
Nocturia, 31, 37, 62, 76, 82
Numbness, legs, 109

Obesity, 26, 56, 68, 109
Oedema, cerebral, 106
    pitting, 2, 4, 12, 37, 58, 88
Oesophagoscopy, 33
Oesophagus, spasm, 25
Onychogryphosis, 90
Osmolality, serum, 32, 68
    urine, 68
Osteoarthritis, hip, 20
Osteomalacia, 57

Pacemaker, cardiac, 36
Pain, abdominal, 4, 15, 17, 37, 41, 45, 49, 54, 56, 62, 68, 80, 84
    back, 17, 56, 109
    calf, 17
    chest, 17, 25, 33, 60, 71, 78, 86, 92, 102
    foot, 98
    hip, 20
    loin, 47
    muscle, 60
    pleuritic, 79, 86, 102
    wrists and ankles, 22
Pallor, 17, 20, 22, 27, 35, 37, 43, 49, 58, 71, 96
Palpitations, 3
Pancreatitis, 85, 91
Papilloedema, 14, 74, 105
Paracetamol overdose, 45
Paraprotein, 109
Peak expiratory flow rate, 14, 51, 52
Pel-Ebstein fever, 71
Percussion note, dull, 2, 4, 22, 66, 75, 86, 88, 102
Pericarditis, 25, 61
Personality change, 106
Petechiae, palatal, 29
    skin, 73
Plantar response, extensor, 5, 9, 39, 64, 94, 105, 109
Plasma cells, atypical, 109
Plasmacytoma, 111
Pneumococcal antigen, 86
Pneumocystis carinii, 107
Pneumonia, 87, 102
Pneumothorax, 52, 78
Polydipsia, 63
    psychogenic, 63, 83
Polyuria, 32, 63, 83
Position sense, impaired, 59
Post-ictal state, 40
Pregnancy, 28
Pressure, intracranial 10, 74, 94, 105
    jugular venous, 2, 12, 75
Proctitis, 54
Prostate, enlarged, 75
Prostate-specific antigen, 75
Proteinuria, 47, 88, 100
Prothrombin time, prolonged, 46, 49, 80
Pseudogout, 99

Pulmonary function tests, 14
    osteoarthropathy, hypertrophic, 23
Pulse, collapsing, 7
    irregular, 2, 20
    slow, 35, 90, 105
Pulses, assymetrical, 17
Pulsus paradoxus, 51
Pus cells, urinary, 37, 47
Pyrexia, 7, 12, 15, 39, 41, 47, 54, 60, 62, 66, 71, 73, 80, 84, 86, 100, 102, 107

Rash, herpes zoster, 92
    macular, 29, 60
    petechial, 73
Reflexes, decreased, 64, 65, 90
    increased, 109
Renal failure, chronic, 37
Retching, 96
Retinopathy, diabetic, 25
Rheumatoid disease, 99
Rigors, 81, 87
Rub, pericardial, 61
    pleural, 86, 102

Salmonella enteritidis, 15
Schilling test, 59
Sclerae, icteric, 49
Shifting dullness, 4, 88
Shingles, 92
Shock, 17, 43, 85
SIADH, 69
Sigmoidoscopy, 54
Skin, reduced turgor, 31
Sodium, urinary, 68, 88
Speech, abnormal, 9, 39, 64, 105
Spider naevi, 4
Spinal cord compression, 110
Splenomegaly, 29, 71, 92
Sputum, blood-stained, 22, 86
    microscopy, 66
    purulent, 12, 66
Staghorn calculi, 37
Staphylococcus aureus, 87
Stiffness, neck, 9
Stokes-Adams attack, 35
Stomatocytes, 5, 66
Streptococcus faecalis, 8
    pneumoniae, 86
Stroke, 65
Subacute combined degeneration, 59
Subdural haematoma, 94
Swallowing, abnormal, 33
Sweating, 7, 17, 20, 25, 37, 47, 66, 71, 73, 80, 87, 93, 100
Swelling, abdominal, 4
    ankle, 2, 4, 12, 33, 49, 58, 75
    generalized, 88
    neck, 2, 71
    toe, 98
Synacthen test, 68

Syncope, 36

Tachycardia, ventricular, 35
Tenderness, abdominal, 37, 45, 54, 62, 80, 84
    epigastric, 20, 56, 96
    renal angle, 47
Tendon reflexes, brisk, 2, 5
Thirst, 31, 62, 82
Thrombocytopenia, 6, 59
Thrombolysis, 26
Thrombosis, cerebral, 65
    deep vein, 102
Thyroid, antibodies, 2
    function tests, 2, 57, 58, 88
Thyrotoxicosis, 3, 23, 28
Thyroxine-binding proteins, 89
Todd's paralysis, 40
Tongue, sore, 58
Tophi, 99
Toxoplasmosis, 30, 72
Tracheal deviation, 49
Transfer, carbon monoxide, 14
Tremor, fine, 2
    flapping, 5, 12
Tuberculosis, 23, 66, 72, 100, 102
Tumour, cerebral, 105

Ulcer, duodenal, 43
    oral aphthous, 54
Ulcerative colitis, 55
Uraemia, 32, 37, 43, 62, 68, 75, 82, 84, 90, 98, 100
Uric acid, serum, 98
Urinary frequency, 47, 76
    incontinence, 31, 39, 77
Urine, dark, 41, 49, 80
Urobilinogenuria, 41
Urogram, intravenous, 38, 47

Ventilation-perfusion scan, 104
Vibration sense, impaired, 59, 109
Vitamin B_{12}, 58
Vocal resonance, reduced, 4, 78
Vomiting, 15, 25, 37, 41, 68, 75, 80, 84, 94, 96, 101

Weakness, generalized, 2, 68, 71
    lateralized, 9, 39, 64, 94, 105
    legs, 22, 59, 109
Weight loss, 2, 4, 22, 33, 49, 54, 56, 66, 71, 82, 87, 93, 100, 107
Wheeze, 12, 51
Wilson's disease, 5

Xanthochromia, 11

Ziehl-Neelsen stain, 67